Rethinking Psychiatry

From Cultural Category to Personal Experience

ARTHUR KLEINMAN, M.D.

THE FREE PRESS

NEW YORK

THE FREE PRESS
A Division of Simon & Schuster Inc.
1230 Avenue of the Americas
New York, NY 10020

First Free Press Paperback 1991

Manufactured in the United States of America

10   9   8   7   6

Library of Congress Cataloging-in-Publication Data

Kleinman, Arthur.
    Rethinking psychiatry.

    Bibliography: p.
    1. Psychiatry, Transcultural. 2. Psychiatry–
Philosophy. 3. Anthropology. I. Title, [DNLM:
1. Cross-Cultural Comparison. 2. Psychiatry. 3. Psycho-
pathology. 4. Socioeconomic Factors. WM 31 K64r]
RC455.4.E8K57   1988   616.89   80-60855
ISBN 0-02-917442-2

To Peter, Anne, Marcia, and Stephen, for whom, after so many years, I have felt the need to explain what my work is about. To Leon, who critiqued what I first wrote, saving me once again from inveterate faults; and who continues to model for me, long after I have formally been his student, the best possibilities for social scholarship in psychiatry. And as always to Joan, for giving me, over almost a quarter of a century, the self-sustaining understanding that what I had to tell was worth saying and therefore worth time and passion.

Realism, like reality, is multiple and evanescent, and no one account of it will do.

Nelson Goodman,
Notes on the well-made world

The biological and the social are neither separable, nor antithetical, nor alternatives, but complementary. All causes of the behavior of organisms, in the temporal sense to which we should restrict the term *cause*, are simultaneously both social and biological, as they are all available to analysis at many levels. All human phenomena are simultaneously social and biological, just as they are simultaneously chemical and physical. Holistic and reductionist accounts of phenomena are not "causes" of those phenomena but merely "descriptions" of them at particular levels, in particular scientific languages. The language to be used at any time is contingent on the purposes of the description. . . .

R. C. Lewontin, Steven Rose,
and Leon J. Kamin,
Not in Our Genes

Contents

Preface

For many psychiatrists, including those in positions of authority within the profession, cross-cultural research is merely exotic. The reality of mental illness in different societies, as depicted in the work of anthropologists and psychiatrists who are engaged in cross-cultural studies, is seen, in North American and Western European psychiatry, as marginal to the purposes of the field. The concept of culture is treated in most psychiatric textbooks as unessential to mental illness and psychiatric treatment. Neither fish (biology) nor fowl (psychology), social norms and cultural meanings simply don't count for much. In the main-line professional ideology, they are "soft." That is to say, the entire cultural apparatus of language, symbols, and interpretations is the source of great ambivalence for the contemporary psychiatric researcher. If cited at all, and most frequently they are not, cultural issues are placed at the bottom of a long list of potentially influential forces; the sheer length and atomized nature of the list dilute the significance of each of its constituents, lending a sense of impracticality and irrelevance to the relationship of culture and mental illness. The present period of biological revanchism in psychiatry—when many psychiatrists seem to believe that understanding the biological basis of mental disorders is, if not around the corner, at most two or three streets away, and that such knowledge will be all the clinician needs to know to treat patients with schizophrenia and depression—is particularly deaf to cultural themes.

One must ask, why should a discipline whose roots are so deeply planted in Western culture, whose major figures are almost entirely European and

xi

North American, and whose data base is largely limited to the mainstream population in Western societies, why should so strongly Western-oriented a discipline regard cross-cultural research among the more than 80 percent of the world's people who inhabit non-Western societies as marginal? Is not cross-cultural research essential to establish the universality of mental illness and the international validity of psychiatric categories? Are not comparative studies an antidote to professional ethnocentrism? Can psychiatry be a science if it is limited to middle-class whites in North America, the United Kingdom, and Western Europe? Yet, in spite of these powerful reasons for international research, psychiatry has made only the slightest of contributions in international medicine, and most psychiatric journals and textbooks evidence little if any interest in the psychiatric aspects of international health.

Against this disquieting background, I will highlight a quite different point of view, a vision of psychiatry in the perspectives of other, non-Western cultures—so huge a portion of humanity, yet so silent a presence in psychiatry. What happens when we make the cross-cultural findings of psychiatric research central to our interpretations of mental illness, or when we make psychiatry the subject of anthropological inquiry? Let us then, place psychiatry in the middle of a ring of mirrors held up by Chinese, Japanese, Indian, Nigerian, Iranian, Melanesian, Hispanic American, and still other cultures' indigenous conceptions, illness perceptions, and therapeutic experiences. The mirrors expose psychiatry's central assumptions and paradigms of practice to cross-cultural comparison. Anthropological studies further extend this revealing cultural analysis into the house of psychiatry itself—its institutions, roles, system of training, and knowledge. To accomplish this task, I ask seven anthropological questions about psychiatry's cross-cultural findings and also about psychiatry's taxonomy and practices. These are not the only questions one might ask, but they are the ones whose discussion I believe is most revealing.

This book was written for the general psychiatrist and for members of that great penumbra of health and mental health professionals that surrounds psychiatry, as well as for the informed layperson who is interested in mental illness and the psychiatric profession. I wrote these chapters not as a scholarly study, but as an account of my thoughts in the course of pursuing cross-cultural and anthropological research for the past two decades. A researcher spends his days in the narrow, twisting streets of a highly technical problem framework; he travels an unmapped, difficult route of minute empirical details that have spun off from the research quest (the broad boulevards) that first motivated his work. Over time that project takes on a life of its own, so that the researcher, in collusion with like-minded colleagues, gets caught up in problems that would seem to anyone but his small research circle remote from the original concerns that prompted the project in the first place. The little roads don't turn back into the major highways; they get even narrower. We end up writing for each other. Every once in a while it is essential to ask what does it all mean? What relevance does our work have to the diverse interests of a wider audience? The seven questions that I have posed represent an effort to work my way back to the original interests that led me into anthropology and cross-cultural psychiatry. Those early interests arose from a desire to rethink psychiatry. That is what I have tried to do in this book, without too much detail, without jargon, and in a space small enough to be encompassed in an evening or two's reading.

The title may seem presumptuous. This is after all not a definitive review of psychiatry that marches chapter after chapter through the chief themes, controversies, and empirical findings. Far from it. I have produced a rather personal essay about a small corner of the discipline, cross-cultural research and its anthropological interpretation—a cameo, not a panorama, a small well-tended garden, not a vast, sprawling park. Yet I feel certain my subject is a microcosm of core tensions in psychiatry broadly. Each of the questions initiates a chapter treating a highly specific, technical problem in cross-cultural research. Through an exploration of that problem, however, the subject is enlarged to touch at least one and usually several abiding controversies in psychiatry. At the end I wish to have created a special vision of psychiatry—not a major canvas, not even a representative picture, and certainly not the only anthropological vision, but one that I have worked toward over years of mastering a special subject and traveling a road few mental health professionals travel.

The view of Florence is distinctive if seen after climbing San Miniato or hiking to Fiesole. The experience of getting there shapes the perception of the vista. No less so for a profession, a clinical practice, a science in the making. This is where my work has taken me. This is what I have seen. This is what troubles me. A different window, to be sure. An unusual angle, granted. A special view, all right; yet one that says something different about questions too often taken for granted or even denied. Each practitioner in the course of a career rethinks his discipline. Here is how psychiatry looks when an anthropologist-psychiatrist who has spent much of his research career in East Asia mulls over his work, reconsiders his readings, and tries to make sense of the major cross-cultural issues in psychiatry as they pertain to the discipline as a whole.

The ideas presented in this book were developed in close collaboration with colleagues in the Harvard medical anthropology and cross-cultural psychiatry group. I wish to acknowledge in particular the formative contribution of my colleague Professor Byron Good—I cannot establish where his ideas leave off and my own begin—and that of other present and former members of our group: Drs. Mary Jo DelVecchio Good, Mitchell Weiss, Peter Guarnaccia, Paul Cleary, Pablo Farias, Thomas Csordas, Janis Jenkins, Linda Garro, and especially Joan Kleinman. Graduate students in anthropology have also contributed to the ideas developed below: Paul Brodwin, Terry O'Nell, John Russell, Scott Davis, Anne Becker, Karen Stephenson, Lawrence Cohen, and Paul Farmer. I wish to acknowledge as well the contribution of foreign visitors in the 1985–86 academic year: Drs. Ravi Kapur (India), Liu Shixie (China), Joan Anderson (Canada), and Rob Barrett (Australia). Support from the Rockefeller Foundation, from an NIMH contract to review cross-cultural studies of depression and anxiety, and from an NIMH training grant in clinically applied anthropology were instrumental in facilitating review of the relevant cross-cultural literature. The cases from China that I describe come from research supported by the Committee for Scholarly Communication with the People's Republic of China of the National Academy of Sciences. A magical month at the Rockefeller Foundation's Bellagio Study Center gave, along with great quiet and enchantment, time and freedom from other responsibilities to revise the text and reconsider the recommendations of colleagues and friends and a wise senior editor, Laura Wolff. The calm competence and genuine humanness of my assistant, Joan Gillespie, made the labor of writing and rewriting much less trying than it otherwise would have been. Finally, my thanks go to the chairmen of the three departments at Harvard of which I am a member—Professors Stanley Tambiah and Irven DeVore (Anthropology), Myron Belfer (Psychiatry at the Cambridge Hospital), Leon Eisenberg (Social Medicine)—for their continuing support of my effort to build a colloquy between anthropology and psychiatry.

Arthur Kleinman
Cambridge
October 1987

Prologue: Why Anthropology?

No anthropologist, in fact, is to be found willing to surrender the abstract world of history for the abstract world of science, to adopt (that is) a purely quantitative conception of man and of society, of civilization, moral development and religion, and to be content with measurements in place of historical events, statistical inference in place of historical fact, statistical generalization in place of historical enumeration. And the reason for this is, perhaps, that the conclusions of such a science would be relatively unimportant.

Michael Oakeshott,
Experience and its Modes

Psychiatry has been overtaken in the 1980s with a fervor for biological explanations. The discovery and development over two decades of psychoactive medications with specific effects on particular disorders spurred research into their physiological effects and in basic neuroscience. The latter is in a "golden" period, with so many breakthroughs occurring so quickly that the entire shape of the research enterprise has changed several times. The medical model with its emphasis on delineating discrete diseases and their equally specific pathological underpinnings, which had been under serious assault from psychodynamic, behavioral, and community orientations, has come back with a vengeance well expressed by the "return to our medical roots" motto.

This in turn has transformed psychiatric epidemiology from a marginal discipline concerned with measuring symptoms of general distress and avoiding the taxonomic chaos of an earlier period into a robust program of disease-specific studies closely tied to the impressive development of research diagnostic criteria, standardized clinical assessment instruments

1

that yield high rates of inter-rater reliability, and a new official diagnostic system of the American Psychiatric Association that has had tremendous influence throughout the profession and worldwide. The latter, DSM-III, sets out operationalized inclusion and exclusion criteria for each of the psychiatric disorders. The growth of psychiatric epidemiology has further clarified the distinguishing characteristics of mental illness and opened up opportunities for remarkably innovative research into the genetic and other neurobiological causes of disease. Although research has thus far failed to identify a unique pathophysiology for each of the psychiatric disorders and although biological "markers" are few and far between, enough progress has been made on the physiological correlates of major depression, panic disorder, and schizophrenia to justify the dominant paradigm of heterogeneous disorders with specific biological sources. Research is now able to establish more reliable rates of psychiatric disease, and to examine vulnerability and provoking factors that place individuals at higher risk.

With all these developments on the biological side of psychiatry, the reader may well ask, why is anthropology at all revelant?

To begin with, the very developments just reviewed also disclose that more is involved in the causal web of psychiatric disorders than changes in neurotransmitters and endocrinological activity. Epidemiological research has begun to parse the social contribution to vulnerability for mental illness through delineation of such factors as life events that are perceived as stressful; social supports that can be assessed as inadequate; and the social origins of helplessness and of a negative sense of self. Family expressions of hostile, negative, and overinvolved emotional response to schizophrenic members have been found to be valid predictors of relapse and worsening course. Cognitive behavioral measures of personal inefficacy and persistent sense of threat and loss have been shown to correlate strongly with depression and anxiety disorders; even more importantly, they have led to the development of psychotherapeutic treatment techniques that are as effective as antidepressants and antianxiety medications. Moreover, unemployment, poverty, and powerlessness continue to show a statistical association with higher rates for most mental disorders. Thus, social psychological aspects of illness and treatment have also been shown to be of considerable significance.

Cross-cultural studies have contributed to this picture. They reveal that the core psychiatric disorders can be diagnosed in a wide range of societies. Certain of these disorders—e.g., depression and anxiety disorders—have particularly high rates in situations of uprooting, refugee status, and forced acculturation. Remarkably, yet still without adequate explanation, the course of schizophrenia has been shown to be better in less technologically developed societies and worse in the most technologically advanced ones. Some disorders appear to be found only in particular culture areas—the so-called culture-bound disorders. These culture-bound syndromes include not just *susto, latah, amok,* and other "folk" illnesses in the non-Western world, but quite possibly agoraphobia and perhaps also anorexia nervosa in the West and among the Westernized elite in developing societies. Patterns of seeking help for psychiatric disturbance vary widely across ethnic boundaries. Some cultures appear to innoculate their members against particular disorders, e.g., alcoholism among Chinese, who until very recently have had extremely low rates, while others put their members at especially high risk, e.g., alcoholism among North American Indians. And of course treatments vary greatly across societies. Research on genetic predisposition, on the family's contribution to the genesis of psychopathology, and on the contribution of environmental factors such as tropical diseases, natural catastrophes, and occupational hazards have all encouraged cross-cultural investigations. Anthropologists have been asked to collaborate in this comparative research enterprise, and a number have done so.

It would be easy to embellish this line of reasoning to establish as practical the use of cultural analysis in psychiatry. But I seek to advance a different justification. Culture holds importance for psychiatry, in my view, *principally* because it brings a special kind of criticism to bear on research regarding mental illness and its treatment. From the cross-cultural perspective, the fundamental questions in psychiatry—how to distinguish the normal from the abnormal; how disorder is perceived, experienced, and expressed; why treatments succeed or fail; indeed the purposes and scope of psychiatry itself—all are caught up in a reciprocal relationship between the social world of the person and his body/self (psychobiology). For the anthropologist, the forms and functions of mental illness are not "givens" in the natural world. They emerge from a dialectic connecting—and changing—social structure and personal experience. That dialectic is the golden thread running through ethnographies of life in different cultural systems, and also through the structure of criticism that anthropologists draw upon to understand mental illness and the mental health professions. In the anthropological vision, the two-way interaction between social world and person is the source of thought, emotion, action.[1] This mediating dialectic creates experience. It is as basic to the formation of personality and behavior as it is to the causation of mental disorder. Mental illnesses are real; but like other forms of the real world, they are the outcome of the creation of experience by physical stuff interacting with symbolic meanings.

The tie between social and personal worlds is mediated by language, symbols, value hierarchies, and aesthetic forms that are the pervasive cultural apparatus which orders social life. Nor is psychiatry exempt from this dialectic. Psychiatric concepts, research methodologies, and even data are embedded in *social systems.* The work of the practitioner and the powers of the profession originate in the same dynamic systems of values and relationships and experiences. Through them, psychiatric diagnostic categories are constrained by history and culture as much as by biology. Indeed, in the concepts of anthropology, biology, history, and culture are deeply interwoven.

In the chapters that follow I will apply this framework of cultural criticism to psychiatric research and practice. The attempt to apply psychiatric categories, so profoundly influenced by Western cultural premises, to non-Western societies is dramatically illustrated in cross-cultural research, the subject of the first three chapters.

Chapter 1

What Is a Psychiatric Diagnosis?

―――――――◆―――――――

Disease is not a fact, but a relationship and the relationship is the product of classificatory process. . . .

Bryan S. Turner,
The Body and Society

What other taxonomies might revolutionize our view—for taxonomies are theories of order?

Stephen Jay Gould,
Animals and us

Individuals are types of themselves and enslavement to conventional names and their associations is only too apt to blind the student to the facts before him. The purely symptomatic forms of our classifications are based on the expressive appearances that insanity assumes according to the temper and pattern of the subject whom it affects. In short, individual subjects operate like so many lenses, each of which refracts in a different angular direction one and the same ray of light.

William James, cited in Eugene Taylor:
William James on Exceptional Mental States,
The 1896 Lowell Lectures

I am sitting in a small interview room at the Hunan Medical College in south central China. It is August 1980 and the temperature is over 100 degrees. I am sweating profusely and so is the patient I am interviewing, a thin, pallid, 28-year-old teacher at a local primary school in Changsha whose name is Lin Xiling.[1] Mrs. Lin, who has suffered from chronic headaches for the past six years, is telling me about her other symptoms: dizziness, tiredness, easy fatigue, weakness, and a ringing sound in her ears. She has been under the treatment of doctors in the internal medicine clinic

5

of the Second Affiliated Hospital of the Hunan Medical College for more than half a year with increasing symptoms. They have referred her to the psychiatric clinic, though against her objections, with the diagnosis of neurasthenia.[2] Gently, sensing a deep disquiet behind the tight lips and mask-like squint, I ask Mrs. Lin if she feels depressed. "Yes, I am unhappy," she replies. "My life has been difficult," she quickly adds as a justification. At this point Mrs. Lin looks away. Her thin lips tremble. The brave mask dissolves into tears. For several minutes she continues sobbing; the deep inhalations reverberate as a low wail.

After regaining her composure (literally reforming her "face"), Mrs. Lin explains that she is the daughter of intellectuals who died during the Cultural Revolution while being abused by the Red Guards.[3] She and her four brothers and sisters were dispersed to different rural areas. Mrs. Lin, then a teenager, was treated harshly by both the cadres and peasants in the impoverished commune in the far north to which she was sent. She could not adapt to the very cold weather and the inadequate diet. After a year she felt that she was starving, and indeed had decreased in weight from 110 to 90 pounds. She felt terribly lonely; in five miserable years her only friend was a fellow middle school student with a similar background from her native city, who shared her complaints. Finally, in the mid-seventies she returned to Changsha. She then learned that one of her sisters had committed suicide while being "struggled" by the Red Guards, and a brother had become paralyzed in a tractor accident. Three times Mrs. Lin took the highly competitive entrance examinations for university education, and each time, to her great shame, she failed to achieve a mark high enough to gain admission.[4] Two years before our interview, she married an electrician in her work unit. The marriage was arranged by the unit leaders. Mrs. Lin did not know her husband well before their marriage, and afterward she discovered that both he and his mother had difficult, demanding, irascible personalities. Their marriage has been characterized by frequent arguments which end at times with her husband beating her, and her mother-in-law, with whom they live, attacking her for being an ungrateful daughter-in-law and incompetent wife. Both husband and mother-in-law hold her responsible for the stillbirth of a nearly full-term male fetus one year before.

Over the past two years, Mrs. Lin's physical symptoms have worsened and she has frequently sought help from physicians of both biomedicine and traditional Chinese medicine. When questioned by me, she admits to more symptoms—difficulty with sleep, appetite, and energy, as well as joylessness, anxiety, and feelings that it would be better to be dead. She has an intense feeling of guilt about the stillbirth and also about not being able to be practically helpful to her paraplegic brother. During the past six months she has developed feelings of hopelessness and helplessness, as well as self-abnegating thoughts. Mrs. Lin regards her life as a failure. She has fleeting feelings that it would be better for all if she took her life, but she has put these suicidal ideas to the side and has made no plans to kill herself.

From Mrs. Lin's perspective, her chief problem is her "neurasthenia." She remarks that if only she could be cured of this "physical" problem and the constant headache, dizziness, and fatigue it creates, she would feel more hopeful and would be better able to adapt to her family situation.

For a North American psychiatrist, Mrs. Lin meets the official diagnostic criteria for a major depressive disorder. The Chinese psychiatrists who interviewed her with me did not agree with this diagnosis. They did not deny that she was depressed, but they regarded the depression as a manifestation of neurasthenia, and Mrs. Lin shared this viewpoint. Neurasthenia—a syndrome of exhaustion, weakness, and diffuse bodily complaints believed to be caused by inadequate physical energy in the central nervous system—is an official diagnosis in China; but it is not a diagnosis in the American Psychiatric Association's latest nosology.

For the anthropologist, the problem seems more that of demoralization as a serious life distress due to obvious social sources than depression as a psychiatric disease. From the anthropological vantage point, demoralization might also be conceived as part of the illness experience associated with the disease, neurasthenia or depression. Here *illness* refers to the patient's perception, experience, expression, and pattern of coping with symptoms, while *disease* refers to the way practitioners recast illness in terms of their theoretical models of pathology.

Thus, a psychiatric diagnosis is an *interpretation* of a person's experience. That interpretation differs systematically for those professionals whose orientation is different. And other social factors—such as clinical specialty, institutional setting, and, most notably in Mrs. Lin's case, the distinctive cultural backgrounds of the psychiatrists—powerfully influence the interpretation. The interpretation is also, of course, constrained by Mrs. Lin's actual experience. Psychiatric diagnosis as interpretation must meet some resistance in lived experience, whose roots are deeply personal and physiological. The diagnosis does not create experience; mental disorder is part of life itself.

But that experience is perceived and expressed by Mrs. Lin through her own interpretation of bodily symptoms and problems of the self, so that the experience itself is always mediated. Because language, illness beliefs, personal significance of pain and suffering, and socially learned ways of behaving when ill are part of that process of mediation, the experience of illness (or distress) is always a culturally shaped phenomenon (like style of dress, table etiquette, idioms for expressing emotion, and aesthetic judgments). The interpretations of patient and family become part of the experience. Furthermore, professional and lay interpretations of experience are communicated and negotiated in particular relationships of power (political, economic, bureaucratic, and so forth). As a result, illness experiences are enmeshed in and inseparable from social relationships.

When a psychiatric diagnosis is made, these aspects of social reality are implied. Diagnosis is a semiotic act in which the patient's experienced symptoms are reinterpreted as signs of particular disease states.[5] But those reinterpretations only make sense with respect to specific psychiatric categories and the criteria those categories establish. All diagnoses share this characteristic, whether the disorder is asthma, diabetes, hyperthyroidism, or depression. However, the signs of psychiatric disorders are more difficult to interpret for two reasons. They are only in part, and even then only for certain disorders, a result of biological abnormality; and psychiatric complaints overlap with the complaints of other ordinary kinds of human misery, e.g., injustice, bereavement, failure, unhappiness.

A psychiatric diagnosis implies a tacit categorization of some forms of human misery as medical problems. Earlier in Western society, what is now labeled depression, a psychiatric disease, may have been labeled as medical disorder (an imbalance in the body's humors), a religious problem (guilt or sinfulness), moral weakness (acedia), or fate (Jackson 1985, 1987). In traditional Chinese medicine, only madness and hysteria were viewed as mental disorders; other problems which we would now call psychiatric were reinterpreted as either manifestations of medical disorder or life troubles owing to the malign influence of gods, ghosts, and ancestors.

In brief, then, though medical diagnosis is taught to medical students and sometimes practiced on patients as a "natural" activity—meaning that symptoms are said to match "underlying" physiological processes—it is anything but natural. What we take a symptom to be is a cultural matter, as is the assumption that a symptom mirrors a single defect in physiological processes. That assumption is not only cultural but naive. One of the most dependable occurrences in clinical care is the practitioner's inability to draw a precise one-to-one correlation between symptom (an experience) and disease diagnosis (an interpretation within a bounded conceptual system). Patients with endoscopic evidence of active ulcer craters in their stomach may have no pain or other symptoms. Conversely, patients with seriously disabling low back pain often have no demonstrable disease. In fact, even when a nerve root is compressed, neurologists cannot say what it is that causes pain (Osterweis et al., eds., 1987, pp. 123–145). There is no direct measurement of pain independent of its subjective experience, and that experience amplifies or dampens or expresses in unpredictable, idiosyncratic ways the symptom pain. The diagnosis of a structural or functional abnormality tells the practitioner little at all about severity of symptoms, functional impairment, or course and treatment response (Feinstein 1987).

Although diagnosis is said to be based on a "hypotheticodeductive" method, in which practitioners test possible diagnostic categories against the patient's symptom story to determine which diagnosis best explains the account and which can be rejected, McCormick (1986) shows that formal hypothesis testing among competing diagnoses is a great rarity in medical practice. Demystifying diagnosis, this physician reasons that simple recognition—based on knowledge, the conceptual system we have learned to use to order the world, and on practical experience, what we have actually been trained to see and do—is the essence of diagnosis in all branches of medicine. The diagnostic interpretation is a culturally constrained activity (though it is also constrained by brute materiality in experience) in which the practitioner's professional training in a particular taxonomic system for ordering experience renders that experience and its interpretation "natural." "What are we missing," asks the naturalist Stephen Jay Gould (1987, p. 24), "because we must place all we see into slots of our usual taxonomy?" The neophyte clinician frequently demands ever more explicit rules to reliably fit sight into slot; the seasoned practitioner often intuitively knows that the fit is good only insofar as it is therapeutically useful and that what is left out of the slotting of experience may be more useful (and valid) than what is hammered in.

In many societies a psychiatric diagnosis has significance in political and legal arenas. In the former, it may be a reason why someone is judged disabled and found worthy of disability-based welfare support. In the latter, it may alter a citizen's rights and responsibilities. The power of an official psychiatric diagnosis in the modern state derives from its formal status as *the* bureaucratic standard for determining everything from competence to revise a will to access to welfare benefits. Increasingly, contemporary society medicalizes social problems (De Vries et al., eds., 1983). Alcoholism, once a sin or moral weakness, is now a disorder. This is not purely arbitrary. Genetic factors and physiological processes are involved. But those factors and processes need to be regarded in a certain way— say, differently from the way we usually regard blue eyes, baldness, an intolerance of strawberries, or an addiction to pasta—before we call them a disease. The same is true of drug abuse, certain kinds of truancy and delinquency for which children and parents were once held legally responsible to school authorities but which are now relabeled as conduct disorder, and a wide range of the experienced problems of daily living, now called stress syndromes, which to a greater or lesser degree have biological antecedents, correlates, and consequents.

Medicalization—whether seemingly scientifically justified or not—is an alternative form of social control, inasmuch as medical institutions come to replace legal, religious, and other community institutions as the arbiters of behavior. This is not always undesirable. In certain societies medicalization may authorize useful social change that is otherwise politically unacceptable. For example, Stone (1984) has shown that the American disability system has come to medicalize problems of poverty, under- and unemployment, and worker alienation. That is to say, economic downturns, rises in unemployment, and job dissatisfaction translate fairly directly into increased numbers of individuals filing disability claims, usually for chronic, low-grade problems such as back pain that they previously did not perceive as impeding physical functioning (see Osterweis et al., eds., 1987). The disability program has thereby functioned to redistribute income—a tacit arrangement that our society would not expressly authorize. Alternatively, medicalization may trivialize and deny social problems (e.g., dealing with Mrs. Lin as if her problem was simply a psychiatric or medical disorder, and not the darker side of major social transformations in modern China). The use of psychiatric diagnoses in the Soviet Union and elsewhere to label dissidents as ill so that they can be isolated and disciplined in prison hospitals is perhaps the most notorious current instance of the abuse of medicalization; but the medicalization of the killing of schizophrenic patients and the mentally retarded, which was the prototype for the killing of Jews, under the Nazis must surely stand as psychiatry's darkest hour (Lifton 1986).

The Meaning of Psychiatric Diagnosis to the Psychiatrist

In a brilliant volume, McHugh and Slavney (1986), senior psychiatrists at Johns Hopkins Medical School, describe psychiatric diagnosis in a phenomenological idiom that I suspect most psychiatrists would find compelling.[6] They refer to psychiatric disorders as naturally occurring forms of mental experience that can be observed in much the same way that the natural scientist observes the stratigraphy of mountains, the structures of the cell, or the forms of diseased arteries, rashes, and cancers. The problem of psychiatric diagnosis then becomes a question of verification. Are the forms present or not? McHugh and Slavney describe the two kinds of verification that psychiatric researchers struggle to establish in studies of the prevalence, manifestations, course, and treatment response of particular psychiatric disorders—namely, reliability and validity. Reliability they define as "verification of observations"; it is "the consistency with which one can make an observation . . . [it] is demonstrated by the correlation between the results of observers using the same technique to make that observation" (p. 4). Reliability is documented by the inter-rater correlation coefficient for congruence of diagnosis by psychiatrists trained in the same diagnostic methodology and using the same criteria.

Validity, on the other hand, is the "verification of presumptions," i.e., the verification of the psychiatric categories themselves. McHugh and Slavney correctly note that the "reliability of some psychiatric observations is high". That is to say, psychiatrists can be trained so as to make the same observations. But reliability reveals only that the measurement of the observations is consistent. It does not tell us if the observations are valid, i.e., whether a patient does or does not have an abnormal mental state such as delusions or hallucinations. After all, diagnosticians can be trained so that they are consistent but wrong.

For example, suppose ten North American psychiatrists are trained in the same diagnostic assessment technique and employ exactly the same diagnostic criteria. They are each asked to interview ten American Indians who are in the first weeks of bereavement following the death of a spouse. They may determine with 90 percent consistency (that is nine out of ten times) that the same seven subjects report hearing the voice of the dead spouse calling to them as the spirit travels to the afterworld. That is a high degree of reliability of observation. But the determination of whether such reports are a sign of an abnormal mental state is an interpretation based on knowledge of this group's behavioral norms and range of normal experiences of bereavement. Now it just so happens that in many American Indian tribes auditory experiences of the voices of the spirits of the dead calling to the living to join them in the afterworld are an expected and commonly experienced part of the sadness and loss that constitute the process of bereavement. This experience does not portend any dire consequences such as psychosis, protracted depression, or other complications of bereavement. Thus, to systematically interpret these normal auditory experiences in this cultural group as "hallucinations," with all that term connotes of abnormality, is an example of reliability without validity. Yet this is often done. I myself have been asked on four occasions to diagnose American Indian bereaved who were undergoing this culturally normative experience as psychotic, and thereby certifiable, by physicians who had made this invalid inference of hallucinations from normal sensory experience.[7]

The problem lies in the positivist bias of most psychiatrists. For McHugh and Slavney, and most of us who have undergone the empiricist training in medical school, observations are direct representations of reality. A word, e.g., "hallucinations" or "delusions," points to an empirical entity, e.g., "abnormal mental state in the world." Advances in effective psychiatric treatment of specific disorders and recognition that clusters of symptoms and signs have the same prognosis not surprisingly encourage the view that depression, schizophrenia, and phobias are "things" in the real world. The picture is more complex. A word, after all, is a sign that signifies a meaningful phenomenon. That phenomenon, as noted above, exists in a world mediated by a cultural apparatus of language, values, taxonomies, notions of relevance, and rules for interpretation. Thus, observations of phenomena are judgments whose reliability can be determined by consistency of measurements but whose validity needs to be established by understanding the cultural context. Perception is theory-driven. The voice of a dead spouse is a hallucination (meaning abnormal sensory process) among most North Americans, for whose reference group the experience is not normative (though perhaps this is not true for some bereaved children—see Egdell and Kolven 1972; and Balk 1983). But it is a normal experience of bereavement among members of many American Indian tribes. The term "hallucination," when used in its clinical sense to mean an abnormal percept, is an invalid interpretation for these individuals.

Validation of psychiatric diagnoses is not simply verification of the concepts used to explain observations. It is also verification of the meaning of the observations in a given social system (a village, an urban clinic, a research laboratory). That is to say, observation is inseparable from interpretation. Psychiatric diagnoses are not things, though they give name and shape to processes involving neurotransmitters, endocrine hormones, activity in the autonomic nervous system, and thoughts, feelings, and behaviors that show considerable stability. Rather, psychiatric diagnoses derive from categories. They underwrite the interpretation of phenomena which themselves are congeries of psychological, social, and biological processes. Categories are the outcomes of historical development, cultural influence, and political negotiation. Psychiatric categories—though mental illness will not allow us to make of it whatever we like—are no exception.

If the cross-cultural perspective sharply raises the issue of validity, it surely does not resolve how it is to be decided. Clearly, validity cannot be a matter of pure subjectivity or complete relativity: the disease and its experience also constrain what diagnosis is valid. What are the criteria we can pose, then, for validity of diagnostic categories applied cross-culturally (i.e., how will we recognize a valid interpretation when we see it)? What techniques can be specified that are likely to produce cross-culturally valid diagnoses? Anthropology poses the question, but offers only a tentative and quite modest answer: assuring the validity of psychiatric diagnoses should involve a conceptual tacking back and forth between the psychiatrist's diagnostic system and its rules of classification, alternative taxonomies, his clinical experience, and that of the patient, which includes the patient's interpretation. Validity is the negotiated outcome of this transforming interaction between concept and experience in a particular context. Thus, validity can be regarded as a type of ethnographic understanding of the meaning of an observation in a local cultural field.

Let us return to the diagnosis of Mrs. Lin's disorder. For her Chinese internists and psychiatrists, the disorder is neurasthenia—a putative "chronic malfunction" of the cerebral cortex associated with nervousness, weakness, headaches, and dizziness, thought to be common among "brain workers" and to have psychosocial as well as biological causes. But it is held to be a physical illness and therefore neither conveys the marked stigma Chinese attribute to mental illness nor implies personal accountability for the associated physical impairment or emotional distress. The way in which Mrs. Lin presents her symptoms is also influenced by the category neurasthenia, which is not only a technical psychiatric taxonomic entity in China but one widely understood in the popular culture. Mrs. Lin's perception of her symptoms selects out and lumps together those symptoms that are familiar and salient to her, namely the ones that fit the popular blueprint of neurasthenia. This practice is reinforced by the relatives, friends, and practitioners to whom she tells the story of her illness, who attend to and emphasize precisely those symptoms that they expect to be present in the neurasthenic syndrome. Thus, Mrs. Lin's symptom report is already an interpretation and therefore a diagnosis.

For myself, the North American psychiatrist who interviewed Mrs. Lin, neurasthenia was not a diagnostic possibility. Ironically "neurasthenia," a term coined by the New York neurologist George Beard in 1869 to describe a disorder he called the "American Disease" because of its presumed prevalence in the United States, was formally expunged from the American Psychiatric Association's latest official Diagnostic and Statistical Manual, Third Edition (DSM-III), in 1980.[8] It had ceased being an acceptable professional term several decades before. In the same year DSM-III's rejection of the term meant neurasthenia was no longer a disease in the United States, I conducted a study of 100 neurasthenic patients in the outpatient psychiatry clinic at the Hunan Medical College. I showed that most of these patients could be rediagnosed, using a standard North American psychiatric protocol translated into Chinese together with DSM-III diagnostic criteria, as cases of major depressive disorder (Kleinman 1986). But there was a rub. Unlike the great majority of chronically depressed patients, these depressed patients responded only partially to antidepressant medication. Although many of the symptoms associated with depression improved, their chief somatic complaints and medical help seeking ended only when they were able to resolve major work and family problems (Kleinman and Kleinman 1985; Kleinman 1986).

I concluded that there were several ways to explain these findings. Neurasthenia might represent culturally shaped illness experience underwritten by the disease depression. The biologically based disease responded to the "therapeutic trial" of drugs; the illness experience ended only when powerful social contingencies "conditioning" the sick role behavior were removed. Chronic pain and other chronic conditions associated with depression have been shown to have a similar treatment response. Once the illness behavior becomes chronic, treatment of the depression may nor may not remove the symptoms of depression, but the illness behavior persists (Katon et al. 1982). Alternatively, both neurasthenia and depression might be regarded as the products of distinctive Chinese and American professional psychiatric taxonomies. In that sense, the experience that both psychiatric systems mapped might be thought of as a case solely of the psychobiology of chronic demoralization, and the mapping itself as a medicalized turning away from the social sources of human misery. In this alternative formulation, the psychiatric diagnosis does not point toward the solution. Rather it disguises the problem.

Other schools of psychiatrists might interpret Mrs. Lin's case and the 100 cases in the Hunan sample drawing on the diagnostic systems of psychoanalytic, behavioral, or other approaches to psychiatry. The World Health Organization (WHO) sponsors a diagnostic system, the International Classification of Disease, Ninth Revision (ICD-9), which does include neurasthenia as an official diagnosis. Although ICD-9 is not used in the United States, it is used in much of the world. Neurasthenia is no longer widely diagnosed in North America, South America, or Western Europe, but it is still a popular diagnosis in Eastern Europe, China, and several Southeast Asian societies. Furthermore, the symptoms and behaviors neurasthenia labels in those societies, which are much like those described in Beard's classic definition, are still common in the United States, despite the fact that the term "neurasthenia" lacks coherence in the North American popular culture. In the West now, new diagnostic labels are employed which emphasize distinctive aspects of this syndrome: "depressive disorder," "anxiety disorder," "somatization disorder," "chronic pain syndrome," and in the North American popular culture, "stress syndrome." A characteristic of these newer terms is that sometimes they describe syndromes that are predominantly bodily, like neurasthenia in China and in nineteenth-century New York, and other times clusters that are predominantly psychological. The presumption is that psychopathology creates both varieties of symptoms. (In this sense, unlike neurasthenia, these disorders, which imply psychosomatic factors, are not regarded as legitimate physical disorders. For that reason chronic viral disorders, like hypoglycemia and other putative physical disorders a decade ago, are the currently fashionable exemplars of "real" disease used to legitimate psychosomatic conditions.) Both forms of symptoms are common in the West, but the overtly psychological variety is decidedly uncommon in most non-Western societies. This important cross-cultural finding—often referred to in the West ethnocentrically as the *somatization* of mental illness in non-Western cultures—I will return to in the next chapter when I discuss the evidence for cross-cultural differences in psychopathology.

The Category Fallacy

If psychiatrists in the United States were to diagnose North American patients similar to Mrs. Lin as cases of neurasthenia, their decision would be seen by their peers as an invalid anachronism. The reification of one culture's diagnostic categories and their projection onto patients in another culture, where those categories lack coherence and their validity has not been established, is a category fallacy (Kleinman 1977). Obeyesekere (1985) offers a telling example. Suppose, he suggests, a psychiatrist in South Asia, where semen loss syndromes are common, traveled to the United States, where these syndromes have neither professional nor popular coherence. Let us imagine that this South Asian psychiatrist has first operationalized the symptoms of semen loss in a psychiatric diagnostic schedule, translated this interview protocol into English, had other bilingual persons translate it back into the original language to check the accuracy of the translation, adjusted those items that were mistranslated, and then trained a group of American psychiatrists in its use and established a high level of consistency in their diagnoses. Using this schedule, he could derive prevalence data for "semen loss syndrome" in the United States. But would these findings have any validity in a society in which there are neither folk nor professional categories of semen loss and in which semen loss is not reported as a disturbing symptom?

This egregious example of the category fallacy is amusing but deplorable. Regrettably, much of cross-cultural psychiatry has been conducted in a rather similar manner, though with one important difference. By and large, cross-cultural studies in psychiatry are carried out by Western psychiatrists (or by members of the indigenous culture who are trained either in departments of psychiatry dominated by Western paradigms or in the West itself) working in the non-Western world.

Dysthymic disorder in DSM-III, or neurotic depression in ICD-9, may be an example of a category fallacy. Chronic states of depression associated with feelings of demoralization and despair have been prominent in the West since the time of Hippocrates (Jackson 1986). Yet in Chinese and other non-Western societies they have not received a great deal of attention. They are influential in the West, especially for the more affluent members of society. However, dysthymia would seem to be an instance of the medicalization of social problems in much of the rest of the world (and perhaps often in the West as well), where severe economic, political, and health problems create endemic feelings of hopelessness and helplessness, where demoralization and despair are responses to actual conditions of chronic deprivation and persistent loss, where powerlessness is not a cognitive distortion but an accurate mapping of one's place in an oppressive social system, and where moral, religious, and political configurations of such problems have coherence for the local population but psychiatric categories do not. This state of chronic demoralization, moreover, is not infrequently associated with anemia and other physiological concomitants of malnutrition and chronic tropical disorders that mirror the DSM-III symptoms of dysthymic disorder (e.g., sleep, appetite, and energy disturbances). In such a setting, is the psychiatrist who is armed with a local translation of the major North American diagnostic instruments (e.g., the Diagnostic Interview Schedule or the Schedule of Affective Disorders and

Schizophrenia) and who applies these to study the prevalence of dysthymic disorder any different from his hypothetical Bangladeshi colleague studying semen loss in mid-town Manhattan? Clearly, great care must be taken before applying this diagnostic category to assure that its use is valid.

For the psychiatric epidemiologist, it is crucial to distinguish a case of a disorder from a person with distress but no disorder. Depression, after all, can be a disease, a symptom, or a normal feeling. Operational definitions that specify inclusion and exclusion criteria are what enable the epidemiologist to proceed. In making the distinction between distress and disorder, taxonomy can become entangled in its own decision rules. For patients with loss of energy due to malaria, appetite disturbance and psychomotor retardation owing to the anemia of hookworm infestation, sleeplessness associated with chronic diarrheal disease, and dysphoria owing to poverty and powerlessness, labeling these four somatic symptoms and one emotion the diagnostic criteria of major depressive disorder is the difference between becoming a case of the disease depression and an instance where depression is a symptom of distress due to a socially caused form of human misery and its biological consequences. Neither DSM-III nor ICD-9 was created with such problems in mind. But they are applied in such settings. The upshot is both a distorted view of pathology and an inappropriate use of diagnostic categories.

As we shall see in the next chapter, there is overwhelming evidence that certain psychiatric diagnoses are valid worldwide—e.g., organic brain disorders, schizophrenia, manic-depressive psychosis, certain anxiety disorders, and perhaps major depressive disorder. But we have substantial reason to doubt whether other psychiatric diagnoses currently popular in the West—e.g., dysthymic disorder, anorexia nervosa, agoraphobia, and personality disorders—are valid categories for other societies.

There is, however, good justification to apply psychiatric diagnoses with rigor and precision. Certain psychiatric conditions are treatable; and without effective treatment, they lead to pain, suffering, disability, considerable expense, and even death. Effective treatment and prevention require a usable diagnostic system. On the other hand, attempts to create airtight systems of diagnoses are ineffective, costly, and dangerous. Diagnostic systems do have unintended consequences, one of which is to serve bureaucratic interests of social control that may not be healthy for patients. There are also intended consequences of diagnostic systems, such as providing official listings for third-party reimbursement, legal procedures, and disability determinations that go beyond the technical needs of the diagnostician but are essential for the patient and the broader society. Both intended and unintended consequences shape the diagnostic system. For example, DSM-III is so organized that every conceivable psychiatric condition is listed as a disease to legitimate remuneration to practitioners from private medical insurance and government programs.

Perhaps the most useful contribution of cultural analysis to psychiatry is to continually remind us of these dilemmas. Cross-cultural comparison, appropriately applied, can challenge the hubris in bureaucratically motivated attempts to medicalize the human condition. It can make us sensitive to the potential abuses of psychiatric labels. It encourages humility in the face of alternative cultural formulations of the same problems, which are viewed not as evidence of the ignorance of laymen, but as distinctive modes of thinking about life's troubles. And it can create in the psychiatrist a sense of being uncomfortable with mechanical application of all too often taken-for-granted professional categories and the tacit "interests" they represent. There is, thank goodness, an obdurate grain of humanness in all patients that resists diagnostic pigeonholing. Most experienced psychiatrists learn to struggle to translate diagnostic categories into human terms so that they do not dehumanize their patients or themselves. Yet, the potential for failure in this core clinical skill is built into the very structure of diagnostic systems. An anthropological sensibility regarding the cultural assumptions and social uses of the diagnostic process can be an effective check on its potential misuses and abuses. Irony, paradox, ambiguity, drama, tragedy, humor—these are the elemental conditions of humanity that should humble even master diagnosticians.

Chapter 2

Do Psychiatric Disorders Differ in Different Cultures?

The Methodological Questions

. . . but where truth is too finicky, too uneven, or does not fit comfortably with other principles, we may choose the nearest amenable and illuminating lie. Most scientific laws are of this sort: not assiduous reports of detailed data but sweeping Procrustean simplifications.

Nelson Goodman,
Ways of World Making

The Anatomy of Cross-Cultural Research in Psychiatry

An anthropologist reading the literature in cross-cultural psychiatry will quickly convince himself that psychiatrists maintain a strong bias toward discovering cross-cultural similarities and "universals" in mental disorder.[1] This bias should not surprise us. Much cross-cultural research in psychiatry has been initiated with the desire to demonstrate that psychiatric disorder is like any other disorder and therefore occurs in all societies and can be detected if standardized diagnostic techniques are applied. In the late 1960s the WHO began a series of international comparisons of schizophrenics in a wide range of societies with precisely this motive.

The first of these studies, the International Pilot Study of Schizophrenia (IPSS), funded principally by the National Institute of Mental Health, set out to show that there are core symptoms of schizophrenia that cluster into more or less the same syndromal pattern in Western and non-Western, industrialized and nonindustrialized societies (WHO 1973, 1979). The accounts of clinicians working in different parts of the world had repeatedly suggested this hypothesis. To prove it required a methodology in which groups of patients in participating research centers in India, Nigeria, Co-

18

lombia, Denmark, the United Kingdom, the Soviet Union, and the United States were assessed by psychiatrists who were rigorously trained in the use of the same diagnostic instrument (the Present State Examination (PSE), a psychiatric interview schedule developed at the Institute of Psychiatry of the University of London), which had been carefully translated into the local languages. The psychiatrists' assessments showed a high degree of reliability within the centers and across the centers.

The IPSS clearly demonstrated that at each center, using strict inclusion and exclusion criteria, samples of psychotic patients could be assembled who displayed similar symptoms. The IPSS had run into several difficulties, however. First, most of the psychiatric patients who presented at the different clinical centers had to be excluded, since they did not fit the criteria. This suggested the possibility that what the study had accomplished was to use a template to stamp out a pattern of complaints that produced a more or less homogeneous sample whose similarity was an artifact of the methodology. The patients who were excluded from the study were precisely those who demonstrated the most heterogeneity. From an anthropological viewpoint, it is this very group—those who were excluded from IPSS sample—who would be expected to demonstrate the greatest cultural difference. Second, in spite of the homogenizing template approach there were still important cross-cultural divergences. One finding was expected based on the clinical literature: certain symptoms differed in prevalence across the centers. For example, most of the cases of catatonia were in India and Nigeria.

But a rather unexpected finding emerged that ran counter to conventional psychiatric reasoning of the time: the *course* of schizophrenia was better for patients in the less developed societies and worse for those in the industrially most advanced societies. This striking difference between countries, however, took a back seat to the finding that core schizophrenic symptoms could be demonstrated in all the centers. The latter was interpreted as further evidence for the biological basis of schizophrenia, which was invoked to explain the similar pattern in spite of greatly different sociocultural contexts. This, by the way, is a quite typical example of the invocation of biological explanations in psychiatry. Ironically, it is the reverse of the argument evolutionary biologists advance to explain the great diversity of species worldwide (Mayr 1981). There biology is viewed as the major source of variation.*

---

*"There are good biological reasons to question the idea of fixed universal categories. In a broad sense, they run counter to the principles of the Darwinian theory of evolution. Darwin stressed that populations are collections of unique individuals. In the biological world there is no typical plant. . . . Qualities we associate with human beings and other animals are abstractions invented by us that miss the nature of the biological variation." (Rosenfield, 1986, p. 22).

Following the IPSS, the WHO launched, again with quite substantial NIMH support, the far more ambitious Determinants of Outcome Study (Sartorius et al. 1986). This study attempted to begin with a more representative sample of schizophrenic patients in the general population who made their first contact with a health or mental health agency—a measurement of so-called first-contact incidence of schizophrenia. That is, patients were assembled from various professional, administrative, and folk healing agencies in well-surveyed catchment areas, who were attending for the first time during an episode of psychotic disorder that met inclusion and exclusion criteria for schizophrenia. Patients and family members were then interviewed as in the IPSS with the PSE, but also with a more elaborate menu of forms assessing symptomatology, various risk factors, and course of disorder over several years.

This study is important enough to examine the findings in detail, because it is the most rigorous and systematic multicultural comparison ever undertaken to study mental illness (Sartorius et al. 1986). More than 1,300 cases were studied in twelve centers in ten countries, including three centers in India (one being the only rural center in the study) and centers in Japan, Nigeria, Colombia, Denmark, the United Kingdom, and the United States (Rochester and Honolulu). The authors' summary of findings includes the following statement: "The frequency of the use of individual ICD [the WHO's International Classification of Disease, Ninth Revision] subtype rubrics varied from 0 to 65 % of the cases in the different centers. Overall, paranoid schizophrenia was the most commonly diagnosed subtype followed by that of 'other' (undifferentiated) and acute schizophrenic episodes. However, in the developing countries the acute subtype diagnosis was used almost twice as often (in 40 % of the cases) as the diagnosis of the paranoid subtype (in 23 % of the cases). Catatonic schizophrenia was diagnosed in 10 % of the cases in developing countries but in only a handful of cases in the developed countries. In contrast, the hebephrenic subtype was diagnosed in 13 % of the patients in the developed countries and in only 4 % of the patients in developing countries" (p. 16). Here we have three important instances of cross-cultural differences, yet the authors' chief conclusion is, "Patients with diagnosis of schizophrenia in the different populations and cultures share many features at the level of symptomatology . . . " (p. 24). They add that, "Once the existence of broad similarities or manifestations of schizophrenia across the centers was established . . . " (p. 25). The authors are of course correct, they do have evidence of "broad similarities," evidence they choose to highlight. But they also have evidence of substantial differences, evidence they choose to deemphasize.

Take, as another example, the data on annual incidence of schizophrenia. The authors make two calculations—one for a "broad" diagnostic definition of schizophrenia that includes virtually all cases in the sample, and another for a "restrictive" definition based on a computer program

(CATEGO) classification of a subtype called S +. For the former, the rates of new cases of schizophrenia per year per 10,000 population range from 1.5 in Aarhus, Denmark, to 4.2 in the rural catchment area of the Chandighar center in India. For the latter, the more restrictive computer-based definition, the range narrows impressively; it now is from 0.7 in Aarhus to 1.4 in Nottingham (pp. 18–19). The authors interpret these findings by arguing that the application of the restrictive definition is valid because it does not result in such a decreased sample size that there is a loss of statistical significance. They do not address the question of the epistemological significance of scrapping most of a sample that shows heterogeneity in order to work with the most homogeneous subsample. They conclude later in the paper that there is a relatively uniform rate of incidence for schizophrenia across the ten societies. From the perspectives of psychiatric epidemiology and biostatistics this may be a valid conclusion, but from a cultural point of view, it is not. The broad sample, again from the cross-cultural perspective, is the valid one, since it includes all first-contact cases of psychosis meeting the diagnostic criteria. The restricted sample is artifactual, since it places a clinical template on the original population that excludes precisely those cases that demonstrate the most cultural heterogeneity. This analytic methodology effectively transforms population-based data into clinic-based data, just the distortion in the IPSS the Determinants of Outcome Study was meant to correct.

To be sure, the restrictive sample demonstrates that a core schizophrenic syndrome can be discovered among cases of first-contact psychosis in widely different cultures. This is an important finding, frequently repeated by clinicians in single-culture studies. It is not, however, evidence of a uniform pattern of incidence. Indeed, the broader sample is the appropriate one to use to make that determination, and it demonstrates the pattern of incidence is not uniform. The restrictive sample is of most interest to psychiatrists because it demonstrates a narrow range of cultural difference; the broader sample is of most interest to anthropologists because it demonstrates a wide range of cultural variation. The biases of the two disciplines (psychiatry and anthropology) are inverse; and therefore it might be argued that both perspectives are essential complements in cross-cultural research. Other epidemiological studies of schizophrenia exhibit a much more substantial range of difference in incidence and prevalence around the globe, as would be expected of a disorder that appears to have a significant genetic basis (given the wide range of human genetic patterns around the world). The WHO findings based on the restricted sample are atypical and suggest the possible influence of an administrative or methodological artifact.

Several other key instances could be adduced in which the authors of the WHO report review findings that disclose both important similarities and important differences; yet Drs. Sartorius et al. elect to focus principally on the former, the "universals." Finally, these influential investigators reassess the data that support better outcome for schizophrenia in centers in developing societies. They report the crucial fact that this finding holds up even when mode of onset (acute versus insidious), which differs significantly across centers with many more acute onset cases in the developing world, is taken into account.

For several decades this finding has been the single most provocative datum to emerge in cross-cultural research in psychiatry (see Lambo 1955; Rin and Lin 1962; Jilek and Jilek-Aall 1970; Murphy and Raman 1971; Waxler 1977). Enormous effort has gone into research methods to verify it. At each stage, leading psychiatric researchers have played down its significance and expressed the expectation that it would turn out to be an artifact of the methodology. The WHO group is to be greatly commended for establishing the validity of this finding. Readers will be profoundly disappointed, however, if they hope to learn more about its sources or implications. The authors are silent on these points, which strangely enough do not appear to have received detailed investigation in this project called "Determinants of Outcome." That is to say, the most important finding of cross-cultural difference receives scant attention compared to that devoted to the findings of cross-cultural similarity. Hypotheses have been generated about the causes of differential outcome since the late 1960s (Murphy 1968, 1982; Cooper and Sartorius 1977; Waxler 1977). Yet none of these seems to have been tested. In the paper's conclusion, the other findings of cultural differences in mode of onset, symptomatology, and help seeking are deemphasized as well.

In all fairness to the authors, this is the first of the final reports from this long-term outcome study, and later reports may well review the data on cross-cultural differences in more detail. Nonetheless, it would seem appropriate to ask why there is such a systematic bias in interpretation. This question is especially appropriate, since we are not dealing with a single instance of such bias, but rather with a pattern repeated time and again in cross-cultural psychiatric research. The WHO's cross-cultural study of depressive disorders (Sartorius et al. 1983) does much the same thing as do the vast majority of reports by other groups of leading psychiatric investigators.

There is, then, a tacit professional ideology that exaggerates what is universal in psychiatric disorder and deemphasizes what is culturally particular. The cross-cultural findings for schizophrenia, major depressive disorder, anxiety disorders, and alcoholism disclose both important similarities *and* equally important differences. Hence the chief anthropological question (how do psychiatric disorders differ across cultures?) is a necessary addition to the main psychiatric question (how are psychiatric disorders similar across cultures?). Psychiatric research increasingly tends to be dominated by epidemiological and survey assessments which involve large samples and achieve statistically significant results. But compared to traditional clinical assessments and anthropological field work, this research employs relatively superficial assessments of patients. Epidemiologists conduct interviews once or at most several times for a total of no more than an hour or two. Ethnography, in contrast, like psychotherapy, places the anthropologist in very intensive long-term relations with a small number of informants. Also like psychotherapy, it involves relations of trust which, over the course of many months and years of research, lead to the uncovering of deeply personal, subtle, and difficult to obtain findings. Those findings make up in validity for what they lack, because of small sample size and informal interview methods, in reliability. What we need are studies that combine both methodologies; a few such studies, which I will review later on, have already been completed, but they account for a very small proportion of cross-cultural research in psychiatry.

In order to illustrate the difficulties that beset cross-cultural psychiatric studies which lack an anthropological component, let us look at a recent and remarkably frank discussion of problems in the assessment of expressed emotion (EE)—an index particularly of critical comments, hostility, and emotional overinvolvement (excessive protectiveness and intrusive concern), but including positive feelings as well expressed by family members toward the patient—in the WHO's Determinants of Outcome Study. High level of negative expressed emotion in the families of schizophrenic patients, as I have already noted, has been found in England and the U.S. to be a strong predictor of relapse of schizophrenic patients (Vaughn and Leff 1976; Karno et al. 1987). The WHO study sought to corroborate this finding as well as to determine if EE plays a similar role in non-Western cultures. Wig et al. (1987) tested whether EE could be rated for the relatives of schizophrenics in the Chandighar center (India) of the Determinants of Outcome project. The senior author, one of India's preeminent psychiatric researchers, and his colleagues note that there indeed were problems in the evaluation of the quality and intensity of "positive remarks" and "warmth" on the taped record of the Camberwell Family Interview (CFI), the British instrument used in these studies in the West, but none affected the assessment of "critical comments" and "hostility." The interpretation of "overinvolvement" had some problems in the Indian sample, but these were ascribed to technical, not cultural difficulties.

Wig and his coworkers operationalized culture as linguistic differences in content and tonal quality of Hindi and English. Verification was defined as the measure of inter-rater reliability between London and Chandighar centers, and also between individual raters. The authors conclude, "It is evident from these results that the rating of critical comments can be transferred satisfactorily from English to Hindi."

These authors have established the reliability of measuring EE in India. They have not established its validity for Indian culture. Validity, as we have seen, is verification of concepts, not observations. Establishing the validity of this measurement requires the study of what EE—negative and positive, high and low—means in an Indian context. Inasmuch as anthropologists have shown, moreover, that emotion in India (as well as other societies) is communicated nonverbally through posture, gait, facial movements, and dress as well as subtle, indirect verbal displays of etiquette and other salient social metaphors such as offering food and receiving gifts (Nichter 1982; Shweder 1985), can an analysis of EE based entirely on direct expression of "critical," "hostile," or "negative" verbal terms be an adequate method of assessment? Culture creates alternative channels for communicating and distinctive idioms for expressing negative feelings. Evaluation of only the verbal channel and the direct idiom may well underestimate the extent to which Indian families communicate negative EE. In fact, Wig et al. have found that EE measured solely in the verbal mode is lower in Indian than in British or Danish families. (Jenkins, in press, has determined much the same for Mexican Americans, but she reasons that to understand this difference requires interpretation of fundamental differences in the family structure and interpersonal communication styles in societies.) The question remains, is the finding that EE can be measured in India with an instrument developed in London valid? The answer to that question cannot come from a coefficient of inter-rater reliability, but must await a much wider-angled ethnographic study of the context of emotional expression and its meaning in the families of schizophrenic patients in Indian culture. In the meantime, research such as the study we have reviewed may result in misleading conclusions.

What Is the Tacit Model in Psychiatry that Exaggerates Biological Dimensions of Disease and Deemphasizes the Cultural Dimensions of Illness?

Many psychiatrists, when they interpret the findings of international and cross-ethnic studies, draw on a usually tacit model of pathogenicity/pathoplasticity which has become close to a professional orthodoxy. In this model, biology is presumed to "determine" the cause and structure of what McHugh and Slavney call the "forms" of mental disease, while cultural and social factors at most "shape" or "influence" the "content" of disorder. The paradigmatic example given to illustrate this ideological view is paranoid delusions in schizophrenia: the biologically based disease is said to cause the *structure* of delusional thought processes; the system of cultural beliefs is said to organize the *content* of paranoid thinking, here as fear that the CIA is out to harm one, there as fear that the KGB is the culprit. In other words, the structure is the same; only the content changes.

Another classical case recounted by psychiatric researchers is the finding that bodily complaints predominate over psychological complaints in depressive and anxiety disorders among members of non-Western societies, among traditionally oriented ethnic minorities, and among less educated members of the lower socio-economic classes (Leff 1981; Kirmayer 1984). This finding is taken to mean that the biology of depression and anxiety disorders underwrites the inner form of these disorders, but cultural beliefs and values so shape the "expression" of the disease that the bodily complaints come to "mask" the "real" psychiatric disease "underlying" them. Indeed, at one point the term "masked depression" was widely used to indicate this phenomenon.

In this stratigraphic version of the mind/body dichotomy, biology is bedrock (the source of pathogenesis), and psychological and especially social and cultural layers of reality are held to be epiphenomenal (i.e., they are said to exert "merely" pathoplastic effects). They need to be stripped away to disclose the "real" disease underneath. As expressed by the illness/disease distinction, the disease is an entity or object hidden by the illness, which is a cultural dressing: catatonic or somatic or hysterical manifestations of the underlying causal process. Diagnosis, as we have already seen, becomes reductionism, the downward semiotic interpretation of the "signs" of the infrastructure of disease out of "the blooming, buzzing confusion" of illness symptoms. The same old wine in another bottle is the distinction between *endogenous* depression, which is supposed to occur independent of social and psychological influences as an inherited biological disorder, and *reactive* depression, which is supposed to be a response to environment and personal experience. This turns out to be an untenable dichotomy for anyone who examines the evidence, since environmental and personal sources of depression are to be found, if carefully looked for, regardless of the severity of the depression or the burden of genetic predisposition.

The anthropological gaze picks out an alternative model. Depression experienced entirely as low back pain and depression experienced entirely as guilt-ridden existential despair are such substantially different forms of illness behavior with distinctive symptoms, patterns of help seeking, and treatment responses that although the disease in each instance may be the same, the illness, not the disease, becomes the determinative factor. And one might well ask, is the disease even the same?

There is overwhelming evidence in North American society that the social and psychological components of the illness experience of chronic pain are more powerful determinants of disability and return to work than the biological abnormalities, which are nonetheless real enough (Yellin et al. 1980; Stone 1984; Osterweis et al. 1987). For these reasons, a more useful model is one in which biological and cultural processes dialectically interact. At times one may become a more powerful determinant of outcome, at other times the other. Most of the time it is the interaction, the relation-ship, between the two which is more important than either alone as a source of amplification or damping of disability in chronic disorder. That dialectic transforms the physiology of pain and suffering, which becomes inseparable from personal perception and social interaction, just as it alters the perception of social relationships, which become part of the neurology of pain (Lewontin, Rose and Kamin 1984).

The tacit pathogenetic/pathoplastic model is also inadequate for under-standing the culture-bound syndromes. The tendency once again is to in-terpret these syndromes, which are either unusually conspicuous or actu-ally specific to a culture area, as exotic (the viewpoint is always that of the homespun Westerner) illness manifestations of particular undelying dis-eases, e.g., *susto* ("soul loss") in Mexico is taken to be a culturally dressed-up version of good old depressive disorder; semen loss syndromes, once abstracted from their unusual constellation of South Asian cultural beliefs, are basically anxiety disorders; *amok* in Malaysia is merely a homicidal version of the brief reactive psychoses seen in emergency rooms in London and New York; and so forth (cf. Kiev 1972).

The picture is a great deal more complex than these reductionistic equa-tions make it out to be. Carr (1978; Carr and Vitaliano 1985) shows, for example, that amok is a *final common pathway of behavior* along which are shunted various kinds of problems: acute and chronic psychoses of var-ious kinds, to be sure, but also alcohol and drug intoxications, criminal behavior without psychopathology, and the like. Guarnaccia et al. (in press) and Low (1985), among others, demonstrate that *ataques de nervios* among Hispanics—pseudo-seizures, syncopes, and other dissociation states—are not simply conversion disorders as a generation of psychoana-lytically oriented Caucasian psychiatrists treating Puerto Rican patients paternalistically claimed when they renamed *ataques* "the Puerto Rican Syndrome." Instead, these culturally approved behaviors may be anything from a medical disease to a normal aspect of bereavement.

Anthropologists suggest that a more accurate mapping of the experience of culture-bound syndromes is provided by regarding such behaviors as idioms of distress. Nichter (1982) has shown that South Havik Brahmin women in India express distressed emotions, family tensions, and other social problems not through a discursive jargon of psychologically minded terms, but rather through traditional cultural idioms such as dietary pref-erence for certain foods, religious metaphors, and the traditional tropes of Ayurvedic medicine (e.g., humoral imbalance in the body). Good (1977), working in a Turkish town in Iran, describes how the idiom "heart distress" condenses key sources of frustration (e.g., typical conflicts in marriage and family) in a culturally sanctioned mode of expression, heart complaints, that communicates distress in both the sick person's body and social rela-tions. The complaint of heart distress opens up negotiations for change, in marriage, family, and work, among protagonists whose troubling life circumstances are metaphorically articulated by this local idiom. The medical anthropological literature contains accounts of cultural idioms of distress for many of the world's cultures.

Not surprisingly, bodily metaphors predominate (Douglas 1970; Needham 1979). In all societies, the body appears to represent both a rich source of symbols for communicating about the social group or the individual person and a way to express the brute materiality of the experience of many forms of misery, much of it socially caused. Bodily complaints can be metaphors of personal, social, and even political distress (Comaroff 1985; Taussig 1980; Turner 1985). The body expresses social status and relationships through patterns of mutilation, adornment, and socially learned styles of gait, posture, and movement. That culture-bound syndromes represent communicative or rhetorical idioms—which, for instance, alert an inattentive husband or sensitize an overly demanding mother-in-law to the personal plight of a long-suffering wife/daughter-in-law or which give the sufferer a little more leverage in negotiating for a less difficult work situation or help in managing household responsibilities in a time of great pressure—does not mean the complaints are without biological significance. Rubel et al. (1984), for example, demonstrate that victims of *susto* in Oaxaca have higher rates of mortality than matched controls. Again, models of culture-biology interactions relating biomedical and anthropological analyses best account for the data.

Heretofore, theory in cross-cultural psychiatry has been impressively underdeveloped. There is no tradition of critical analysis of alternative models. There has been a tendency to avoid engaging the pertinent scholarly context of ideas in a critical colloquy. Avoidance of theoretical issues may have been useful at an earlier stage in psychiatry, when grand theories abounded and there was little agreement on diagnostic criteria. But it can no longer be justified. Anthropology's contribution is to press for a more theoretically sophisticated and conceptually critical approach to cross-cultural studies, an approach that develops midrange concepts to explain how culture affects mental illness. Translation is a seemingly prosaic but in fact particularly significant issue for advancing a cultural critique of psychiatric research; it suggests alternative concepts and methods of inquiry.

How Does Translation Influence the Study of Mental Illness in Different Cultures?

Medical, including psychiatric, research often proceeds as if translation was a nuisance to be managed in much the same way as one controls the demographics in matched samples. For psychologists, translation looms as a larger concern but one that is reduced to a technical problem in research methods. It can be managed through a rigorous process of translation by one set of bilingual key informants; back translation into the original language of the psychometric instrument by yet another set of bilingual informants; negotiation of the differences in order to restructure the questionnaire to be semantically (not merely lexically) accurate; and testing of its reliability compared to other measures of the same phenomena that have already been used in the recipient society and by different investigators. Quantitative standards, such as a correlation coefficient for reliability, once met, relieve the psychologist's concern about the translatability and utility of her questionnaire in another culture.

For the ethnographer, in contrast, translation is neither a nuisance nor a strictly technical question. Rather, translation is the essence of ethnographic research. In anthropological studies, description of indigenous categories of thought, modes of communication, and patterns of behavior is at heart the translation from one cultural system into another. That translation is what the ethnographer spends her days doing—i.e., getting it right from the native point of view. Having achieved a valid understanding of the local context in its own terms, the ethnographer then undertakes another type of translation in which she puts her findings into terms and categories appropriate for transcultural comparison. That kind of translation is the final, not as in psychiatry the first, step in research. Therefore, the cultural challenge to psychiatry is to take a much more strenuous, systematic, and contextual approach to translation. Ethnographers insist that psychiatrists recognize translation as the central issue in cross-cultural research. A few examples of a cultural orientation to methods of translation used in psychiatric research should clarify why this subject is so important.

Most psychiatric assessment instruments are developed in a vernacular that is quite difficult to translate into other languages. North American diagnostic instruments, for example, frequently depend on colloquial terms like "feeling blue" or "feeling down" to evaluate depressive affect. A strictly lexical translation of these terms would have no meaning in most non-Western languages. Manson et al. (1985) translated the widely used and NIMH-sponsored Diagnostic Interview Schedule (DIS) into Hopi, an American Indian language. One of the DIS questions includes the concepts of guilt, shame, and sinfulness in the same sentence. Each of these concepts was clearly understood to convey distinctive meaning by 23 bilingual Hopi health professionals. They indicated to Manson and his colleagues that three separate questions were required to render this questionnaire item into Hopi without confounding potentially different responses. Kinzie and his coworkers (1982) experienced a similar problem in developing a Vietnamese-language depression scale for use with Vietnamese refugees in the United States. They found that "shameful and dishonored" but not "guilt" discriminated depressed from nondepressed Vietnamese Americans.

When Gaviria et al. (1984) translated the DIS into Spanish for research in Peru, many of the substances listed in the substance-abuse section of the questionnaire were unavailable in Peru; on the other hand, coca paste, a major drug in Peru, did not appear in the North American–oriented DIS. For some of their informants who were illiterate and who had no prior experience filling out a questionnaire, the responses elicited represented a misunderstanding of intentions more than an accurate reflection of their mental state. Gaviria et al. also note that in their experience the responses to an interview relate to theoretical constructs within the local culture. Neurasthenia, as we have seen, is a salient cultural category in the popular culture in China, though it no longer forms a coherent category for most North Americans. For a research interview to be conceptually valid in China, it needs to operationalize this category, turn neurasthenia into a series of linked questions that explore its phenomenology and meaning, not simply list its symptoms. In their entirety, several of the leading symptom checklists commonly used in psychiatric research include the symptoms that appear in the neurasthenic syndrome. Because these are not organized into a syndromal cluster, however, the symptom checklists fail to elicit subjects' informed response. Thus, Chinese research subjects suffering from neurasthenia could not convey, through responses to items in such Western-based questionnaires, either that they had neurasthenia or the full range of their experience of that condition (Kleinman 1982; Cheung et al. 1981). This is true in all non-Western contexts. Unless questionnaires add operationalized symptom clusters for locally salient illness experience, they fail to validly register cultural differences in the symptomatology of mental illness.

Intracultural diversity makes the task of developing culturally meaningful translations even more complex. Canino et al. (1987) used the Spanish-language version of the DIS (developed at UCLA for use with Mexican Americans) in a study of Puerto Ricans. They had to change 67 percent of the questions in order to adapt the instrument to the colloquial Spanish spoken by Puerto Ricans. Level of acculturation, history of migration, education, class, sex, age cohort, and urban/rural residence further influence the process of effective translation. Yet few psychiatric studies go to the trouble to systematically consider these variables. Indeed, I have reviewed grant applications by psychiatrists proposing research with rural populations in South America in which they translated their questionnaires from English into Spanish even though most of their subjects were Indians who were likely to speak Spanish poorly if at all.

To assess cultural differences adequately, it is essential to translate local idioms of distress and add them to standard questionnaires, while deleting those that make no sense in the local culture. This may seem obvious, but it is not routinely done. For example, Ebigbo (1982) has demonstrated that Nigerian psychiatric patients have a unique set of somatic complaints—

"things like ants keep on creeping in various parts of my brain" and "I feel heat in my head"—which are not represented in standard symptom screening scales, including those used in most research with Nigerian patients; yet they are robust predictors of mental illness. Kinzie et al. (1982) found that among Vietnamese Americans, the concept "sadness" was represented by three different terms and "discouragement" by two. Among Latinos, Guarnaccia (personal communication) points out, headaches are described as *dolor de cabeza* ("headache") and *dolor del cerebro* ("brainache"), and these two expressions may be associated with different experiences and disorders. In a number of African cultures, anxiety is expressed as fear of failure in procreation or in dreams or complaints about witchcraft. To adequately evaluate psychopathology among members of these cultures, it is necessary to ask about these fears, dreams, and complaints.

During the 1950s and 1960s, a number of multiethnic psychiatric studies were carried out in New York City (Srole et al. 1962; Dohrenwend 1966; Haberman 1970, 1976) using the 22 Item Scale (22IS) a symptom checklist containing primarily somatic symptoms of anxiety and depression. These studies consistently found that of the ethnic groups in the sample, Puerto Ricans reported the highest number of symptoms. In the Midtown Manhattan Study this finding was especially striking (Srole et al. 1962). Although the Puerto Rican subsample was quite small, 61 percent of the Puerto Rican subjects reported experiencing impairing levels of symptoms compared with 31 percent of the non-Puerto Ricans. Not one of the 27 Puerto Ricans was rated as "well"! Dohrenwend (1966) demonstrated that the differences in reported levels of symptoms were better explained by attitudes toward the social desirability of reporting psychosomatic symptoms than by different levels of psychopathology (see p. 31). Guarnaccia (personal communication) argues that the symptoms of the 22IS fit closely with the category *nervios* ("nerves") among Puerto Ricans, a folk complaint associated with headaches, trembling, palpitations, difficulty concentrating, insomnia, worries, and gastrointestinal symptoms. He suggests what made Puerto Ricans respond so readily to the scale is that the instrument inadvertently tapped a salient cultural category associated with the stress of acculturation of recent Puerto Rican immigrants to New York City—a problem hardly ever mentioned in psychiatric investigations.

There are other means by which culture influences psychiatric research. One of those concerns the repeated finding that bodily states and psychological experiences are monitored (i.e., perceived), assessed, and reported differently by members of different cultural groups. In Zborowski's (1952) classical account of difference in reporting pain among Irish, Italian, Jewish, and Anglo-Saxon Americans, ethnicity correlated highly with degree of expressivity, pain tolerance, and worries over the sigificance of the experience. Angel and Thoits (1987) review evidence indicating that Mexican Americans focus their concern on different parts of the body and different symptoms than the mainstream North American population. "Nerves," for example, is no longer a common complaint among middle-class members of North American society, whereas it is still an important idiom of distress among Hispanics and natives of Appalachia. "Falling out," "high blood," and "pressure" are complaints of lower-socioeconomic-class Southern blacks, based on folk medical beliefs, which are not routinely assessed by psychiatrists or epidemiologists (Snow 1974; Weidman 1977; Nations et al. 1985), even though they are important expressions of distress in this population.

There is evidence, to which I have alluded, that the social undesirability (stigma) of reporting distressing symptoms when asked in questionnaire-based studies is less among Hispanics than among blacks or Northern European Americans (see also, Haberman 1976; Krause and Carr 1978; Vernon et al. 1982). This difference appears to increase the likelihood that Hispanic subjects will be defined as suffering more distress and disease on epidemiological scales. Gaines and Farmer (1986) show that complaining about health and personality problems among impoverished members of Southern European cultures has a long history of providing the status of cynosure to so-called visible saints, individuals who become moral exemplars of the burden of life's difficulties and the obdurate grain of martyrdom in human nature. Complaining in this cultural context is positively valued and rewarded. This is in strong contrast to Northern European traditions that emphasize austerity, continence and understatement of personal troubles and that attach great stigma to the open expression of complaints as an indication of personal "weakness." Thus, different cultural norms influence how individuals in different societies respond to questionnaires. The repeated finding on psychiatric epidemiological surveys that blacks report fewer complaints in spite of suffering high levels of distressing social conditions appears to be part of a long-standing and understandable response strategy by means of which blacks have tried to deflect the prying attention of social agencies. Not surprisingly, then, black respondents give more information to black interviewers (Dohrenwend 1966).

The social setting of research also influences the findings. Subjects interviewed in a medical clinic—where much of the cross-cultural research has been conducted that discloses more somatization of psychological problems in the non-Western world—are more likely to express physical complaints than subjects interviewed in their homes. After all, their expectation is likely to be physical complaints are what physicians want to hear. Mitchell et al. (1985) report another common problem in cross-cultural research. A North American interview schedule which they used with Peruvian Indians was insistent to the point of violating the reticent style of response of Indians when talking to non-Indian professionals. Cultural convention sometimes makes it virtually impossible to ask questions in surveys about sexuality and other highly charged topics. For example, surveys in China frequently drop items about sexuality from the Western questionnaires they employ, for this reason. Yet such information can often be obtained by ethnographers, who develop relationships of trust over long stretches of time with informants that enable them to probe intimate meanings.

From an anthropological vantage point, these potentially confounding cultural influences on the determination of whether a patient in another society or a member of an ethnic minority group should be assessed as ill, and if so with what specific diagnosis, should make psychiatrists extremely cautious in interpreting the results of past surveys and in planning new research. This is an especially important caution for clinicians, since misdiagnosis is commonplace in cross-cultural settings of health care. Nonetheless, in spite of the difficulties I have reviewed, some recent studies have systematically taken into account cultural differences in a way that is a model for future research.

Manson and his colleagues (1985) organized a combined psychiatric epidemiology and ethnography of depressive illness among Hopi Indians. A team of anthropologists and psychiatrists first carried out a systematic translation of a standard psychiatric assessment interview (DIS) into Hopi based on a detailed anthropological understanding of the local context. They then elicited Hopi categories of sickness that are believed to affect people's minds or spirits. From this list they identified five categories of illness which intersected in different ways with the North American category of depressive neurosis. The English translations of these indigenous categories of disorder include "worry sickness," "unhappiness," "heartbroken," "drunken like craziness with or without alcohol," and "disappointment; pouting." The symptoms for these Indian disease concepts were included in the diagnostic instrument developed by Manson, who is himself a Native American anthropologist, and his psychiatric coworkers. "Unhappiness" correlated strongly with depressed affect on the DIS; it did not correlate with any of the other symptoms of depression. "Heartbroken," on the other hand, correlated strongly with a number of the concomitant symptoms of depression. Thus, this interdisciplinary team was able to demonstrate important local expressions of disorder that are not subsumed by existing North American psychiatric categories and that would be missed if research was conducted by following only the standard North American research criteria. Their work is also an excellent model of how to translate and adapt clinical diagnostic interviews and questionnaires so that they are valid in a very different cultural setting. In an earlier study, Carstairs and Kapur (1976), a Scottish psychiatrist raised in India and an Indian psychiatrist trained in Scotland, developed a sensitive psychiatric interview schedule for use in a local area of Karnataka in south India, based on their extensive review of clinical records of patients from that area and knowledge of local idioms of distress. These local symptom clusters and idioms were then built into their diagnostic interview. These studies indicate that culturally sensitive and anthropologically informed psychiatric research is feasible. The extreme relativism of some antipsychiatry anthropologists is as outrageously ideological as is the universalistic fundamentalism of some card-carrying biological psychiatrists.[2]

Chapter 3

Do Psychiatric Disorders Differ in Different Cultures?

The Findings

Even among facts some are more equal than others.

> Jacques Barzun,
> *A Stroll with William James*

. . . close observation of individual differences can be as powerful a method in science as the quantification of predictable behavior in a zillion identical atoms . . . .

> Stephen Jay Gould,
> *Animals and us*

While ideal studies are rare, one can reanalyze the cross-cultural research literature in light of the problems discussed in the preceding chapter and derive some reasonable conclusions as to which findings seem valid and what their implications are.

Epidemiology

The prevalence data (total cases at a particular time) for schizophrenia—a serious mental disorder of unknown cause characterized by delusions, hallucinations, associations of unrelated ideas, social withdrawal, and lack of emotional responsiveness and motivation—indicate a band of prevalence rates ranging from roughly two to ten cases per thousand population across a range of populations (Sartorius and Jablensky 1976). Lower rates have been reported in less developed societies and the highest rates in North

America and certain European societies (Fortes and Mayer 1969; Torrey 1980; Sikanerty and Eaton 1984). Although some incidence data (new cases in a defined period of time) are available for European societies, the data for non-Western societies are very limited and controversial. As we have seen in the World Health Organization studies, there is evidence for a wider range of incidence rates when the broader, heterogeneous sample of schizophrenic patients is used to calculate rates, and a narrower range when the more homogeneous sample is employed. Other studies report small-scale, preliterate societies with hardly any cases of schizophrenia and communities, often small, isolated Scandinavian ones,* with very high rates of schizophrenia (cf. Warner 1985 for the most comprehensive review).

It is hard to know what to make of these findings. They certainly represent a wider continuum than is suggested by the professional catechism that there is a relatively narrow band of prevalence of this psychiatric disorder cross-culturally. There are, furthermore, families that have much higher rates of this major mental illness than most others in the population. Twin studies, including those comparing twins of schizophrenic parents who are adopted out into nonschizophrenic families, indicate that there is a significant genetic basis to this disorder.[1] But the genetic contribution is controversial; most models of the disorder invoke an interaction between social environment, genetic endowment, and neurobiological processes, making for a complex causal nexus. It is clearer to say in 1987 that the cause is unknown, as Carpenter, McGlashan, and Strauss (1977), leading psychiatric researchers who have devoted their careers to the study of schizophrenia, concluded a decade ago. Perhaps the chief epidemiological conclusion is simply the finding of patients with the core symptoms of schizophrenia in a very wide variety of societies. This mental illness is no myth.

Schizophrenia in developing societies is much more likely to present with an acute than an indolent onset; chronic mode of onset is more common in Western societies. DSM-III's diagnostic criteria strictly limit cases of schizophrenia to those that have had a course of at least six months. Acute onset cases that are of less than six months duration are not diagnosed as schizophrenia by the standards of DSM-III. The WHO's ICD-9 does not have this requirement. Thus, different categories and different phenomena interact to create incommensurate findings. Acute onset psychosis of short duration is probably not the same disease as chronic onset long-duration psychosis (Stevens 1987). Whether acute onset and chronic onset psychoses of the same duration are indeed the same disorder is unclear. Schizophrenia is probably a group of syndromes. From the cross-

---

For example, Book et al. (1978) report a rate of 17 cases per 1000 for northern Sweden; and Torrey et al. (1984) report a rate of 12.6 per thousand for a high prevalence area in western Ireland.

cultural perspective, schizophrenia is organized as much by taxonomies as it is by disease processes.

Warner (1985) advances a substantial body of evidence to suggest that the occurrence and course of schizophrenia are strongly conditioned by the political economy. Unemployment and economic depression in the West and the development of capitalist modes of wage labor in non-Western societies appear to lead to greater numbers of individuals manifesting schizophrenia and fewer of them improving. This is a topic to which I shall turn in the next chapter. Warner also explains how analysts of the cross-cultural data base on the prevalence of schizophrenia could come to almost diametrically opposed views of the relative frequency of the disorder in non-Western and Western societies because of ideological commitments which lead psychiatrists to emphasize certain studies while discounting or even ignoring others.

The prevalence data for brief reactive psychosis—an acute psychosis closely associated with a serious stressful life event in a person without premorbid pathology and with recovery within days or weeks without any significant chronic symptoms or persistent disability—show that this disorder constitutes a much larger portion of acute psychoses in nonindustrialized, non-Western societies than in the industrialized West (Langness 1965; Manschreck 1978; Murphy 1982). Psychiatric researchers are concerned that such cases of brief reactive psychosis misdiagnosed as schizophrenia confound cross-cultural comparisons. But for the anthropologist, brief reactive psychoses are of particular interest because they are the one psychotic disorder that has enormously different prevalence rates cross-culturally. Moreover, they show great diversity in form—in an arc running from trance and possession states occurring outside culturally authorized settings to schizophreniform experiences—and such impressive cultural shaping that certain brief reactive psychoses are included in the culture-bound syndrome category. This group of psychiatric disorders is neither well-studied nor given a central place in psychiatry; yet for cultural analysis it is of very special significance. It is not surprising, then, that anthropological studies of individual brief reactive psychoses are more frequent than anthropological studies of schizophrenia. Studies disclose that of all forms of madness brief reactive psychoses bear the strongest causal relationship to immediate life event stressors, especially stressors that are of particular cultural salience, that they are the most culturally diverse of all psychoses, that they overlap with final common pathways of normal behavior (e.g., culturally approved trance states), and that they respond well to indigenous healing systems (Langness 1965; Kleinman 1980; Lewis 1971).

The epidemiology of nonpsychotic disorders around the globe is even more variable. Depression is the best case in point. The findings reveal a much greater range of variation than for schizophrenia. There simply are no studies in the non-Western world, however, comparable in rigor and standardization to the Epidemiological Catchment Area (ECA) studies sponsored by the NIMH in the United States. That set of studies, a particularly expensive undertaking involving investigators trained to use the same interview schedule (DIS), surveyed communities in five sites. Six-month prevalence rates (i.e., total number of cases detected in a period of six months) for affective disorders (chiefly depression) ranged from 4.6 to 6.5 percent. Lifetime prevalence rates (i.e., total number of individuals in the study population who experienced an episode of depressive disease sometime during their life) ranged from 6.1 to 9.5 percent. Major depression, as in earlier research, was found to be more common in women and in urban areas (Blazer et al. 1985; Myers et al. 1984; Robins et al. 1984).

Reviewing the English-language literature for industrialized Western societies, Boyd and Weissman (1981) estimated the point prevalence (number of cases at a particular point in time) of clinical depression (not including manic-depressive disorder, a psychosis) in studies using newer, more reliable diagnostic techniques as 3.2 percent in males and 4.0 to 9.3 percent in females. The range of prevalence in reports from nonindustrialized, non-Western societies is much greater.

Despite reports during the colonial period that depression was uncommon in India, Venkoba Rao (1984) states that recent studies indicate depression is a common disorder, though, because the variation of rates across different cultural areas in India is wide, he is uncertain just how common. Rao cites Indian rates of 1.5 to 32.9 per thousand in the general population. Among the highest rates currently reported are those for Africa: 14.3 percent for men and 22.6 percent for women in Uganda (Orley and Wing 1979). Ironically, an earlier generation of colonial psychiatrists, many of whom were paternalistic and racialist, claimed that depression was rare in Africa, India, and other non-Western culture areas owing to putative weaknesses in the cognitive and affective states of indigenous populations.[2]

Increased rates of depression in Africa and other non-Western cultures appear to be the result of the use of more culturally appropriate diagnostic criteria and standardized research methods in studies that sample the general population and therefore do not rely, as did an early generation of studies, on clinic-based figures that are biased by different patterns of help seeking. But Prince (1968) and H.B.M. Murphy (1982, p. 143) suggest, in addition to correction of methodological shortcomings, there has probably been a general increase in rates of depression in many non-Western societies due to the pressures and problems of modernization. Clearly, the finding of high rates of depression in Uganda must, at least in part, reflect the political chaos and murderous oppression that the members of that society have so tragically experienced.

Lin and Kleinman (1981) reviewed the epidemiological studies of mental illness in China since the early 1950s, which include some of the largest population surveys ever attempted, involving tens of thousands of respondents. They found that prior to 1981, with the exception of manic-depressive psychosis and involutional melancholia, a psychosis among the elderly, clinical depression was simply not reported. In the past few years the Chinese have begun to publish clinic-based studies that record higher rates of depression (an increase from 1 percent to 20 percent of outpatient samples), though rates still lower than in the West (see studies cited in Kleinman 1986). This increase is almost certainly the result of using newer Western-influenced diagnostic criteria and psychometric assessment tools. The WHO's comparative international study of *Depressive Disorders in Different Cultures* (Sartorius et al. 1983), a multicultural project involving centers in Japan, Iran, and other non-Western societies, does not cite prevalence rates among its findings. Tsung-yi Lin and his colleagues in Taiwan (1969) reported a great increase in the rates of neuroses including depression from the time of a first survey of three communities in the late 1940s to a second survey, conducted by the same research team with the same criteria and methods, 15 years later, during the period of Taiwan's rapid modernization. Clinicians in many non-Western societies have claimed similar increases, but pre- and post-epidemiological surveys, like Lin's, are few in number. There is a strong possibility that, at least in some societies, the norms and idioms for expressing distress have changed so substantially that the expression, not necessarily the occurrence, of depression is more common. We do know, however, that the rates of depression and other neurotic conditions are elevated in refugee, immigrant, and migrant populations owing to uprooting, loss, and the serious stress of the acculturation process (Beiser 1985, Beiser and Fleming 1986). Selective uprooting of those most vulnerable to mental illness does not play a significant role in forced migrations of the most recent Southeast Asian and South American refugees in North America, so that the data on refugees probably are an accurate reflection of psychiatric casualities of uprooting and acculturation.[3] Furthermore, at least in North America, leading psychiatric epidemiologists claim to have incidence data that the rate of depression among young adults is on the rise (*Psychiatric News* 15 May, 1988).

Some advance has also been made in understanding risk factors for depression. In a classic study, Brown and Harris (1978) convincingly demonstrated that among working-class women in England, relative powerlessness, absence of affective support, and the social pressures of child rearing and no job outside the home significantly increased their vulnerability to serious life event stressors, like loss; those with marginal self-esteem were pushed over the edge into generalized hopelessness and clinical depression. Kleinman (1986) has found the same pattern of vulnerability and provoking agents among Chinese depressives, though the particular sources of their vulnerability differ. Good, Good and Moradi (1985) reported comparable findings among Iranian immigrants in the United States. Beiser (1987) has identified a mediating process in depressed and anxious Southeast Asian refugees to Canada: excessive nostalgia and preoccupation with self-perceptions of time past as ideally positive and future time as threatening and undesirable identify those at highest risk for developing distress at a later date. The causes of differential susceptibility remain a very important subject for cross-cultural comparisons.

For the other neurotic disorders, there is terribly little valid cross-cultural epidemiological data. In earlier epidemiological studies, either anxiety was mixed in with other neuroses or the criteria for distinguishing it from other disorders were not enumerated. In an earlier review of what cross-cultural literature does exist, my colleague Byron Good and I (1985) estimated that, with the exception of studies of Australian aborigines, anxiety disorders are diagnosed at a rate of 12 to 27 cases per thousand population. In the ECA studies, six-month prevalence rates of anxiety and somatoform (somatization disorder, hypochondriasis, psychogenic pain) disorders varied from 6.6 to 14.9 percent and lifetime rates from 10.4 to 25.1 percent (with differences largely due to different rates for phobias), making this combined category the commonest psychiatric condition in the United States. Iranian studies described prevalence rates of 27 and 8 per thousand in one project for anxiety disorders among villagers and city dwellers, respectively, and 48 and 38 per thousand for a mixed category of anxiety and somatoform disorders in another. Indian studies cite rates of 17.8, 20.5, and 12 per thousand population for the same category.

The studies of Australian aborigines are a marked contrast. Population surveys of 2,360 individuals turned up only one case of "overt anxiety" (Jones and Horne 1973). The Cornell-Aro Mental Health Project in Nigeria conducted by the psychiatrist-anthropologist Alexander Leighton and his colleagues (1963b) reported high levels of anxiety symptoms (this study did not make disease designations) in village and town residents, 36 and 27 percent, and found high levels of respondents who were significantly impaired, 19 and 16 percent. By contrast, the Sterling County study in Nova Scotia by the same team of investigators (Leighton el al. 1963a) found far fewer anxiety symptoms (13 and 10 percent) but twice the rate of impairment (38 and 32 percent). As with their findings for depression, Orley and Wing's (1979) comparison of Ugandan village women and London women found higher rates of anxiety disorders in the former. (Given the high rates of infectious diseases, many undiagnosed, among rural dwellers in the non-Western world, it is extremely difficult to know what to make of attempts to diagnose their anxiety and somatoform disorders.) Many researchers of the common culture-bound syndromes—especially fright and soul loss disorders, neurasthenia, and *taijinkyofusho*, a Japanese phobic reaction associated with fear of others—hypothesize that these conditions may represent culturally authorized final common behavioral pathways for anxiety disorders (Carr and Vitaliano 1985; Simons and Hughes, eds., 1985). Consequently, the cross-cultural epidemiological literature on depression and anxiety disorders indicates that these are common around the globe, particularly in patients in general medical clinics, though precise determination of comparative rates is not feasible at present and reasons for the wider cross-cultural disparities are uncertain.

Studies also generally show that these disorders are found at higher rates among women (though several studies show the reverse) and members of lower socioeconomic classes in a number of societies. The most recent studies of depression and gender have supported Brown's model of the effect of powerlessness and low self-esteem on the etiology of depression in women (Finkler 1985; Kleinman 1986; Good and Kleinman 1985; Lock 1986, 1987; Gaines and Farmer 1986). The definitive epidemiological data is not in, but women and certainly poor women appear to be at higher risk for mental illness in a number of societies.[4] For the major mental disorders, the social context, which I review in Chapter 4, appears to be the chief source of cross-cultural diversity. But this is in part because genetic, temperament, and other biographical variables, which might explain why only some individuals exposed to the same pressures become ill, have not been systematically studied outside the Western world.

That research on American Indians and Hispanic Americans shows both very high and quite low rates in different studies warns us again of the importance of intracultural diversity. The association of depression with high rates of alcoholism in some (but not all) American Indian and Alaskan Native populations emphasizes as well the potentially important relationship between alcohol abuse and mental illness. For example, in the ECA studies, lifetime prevalence rates for substance abuse ranged from 15 to 18 percent with alcoholism 11.5 to 15.7 percent, and 15 percent of those with alcoholism had depression (Robins et al. 1984). Alcoholism rates are rising in a number of areas around the world, though, as Heath (1986) sagely cautions, the evidence for a worldwide epidemic, which some mental health professionals claim is happening, is simply not there. Nonetheless, alcohol rates in East Asian societies (Japan, Hong Kong, Taiwan, even China), which were traditionally very low by Western standards, are now increasing, and this will complicate the cross-cultural epidemiology of mental disorders very considerably, because it will be necessary to determine if changes in rates of psychopathology are due to alcoholism (Lin and Lin 1984).

Our original question was, do psychiatric disorders differ cross-culturally? The epidemiological rates indicate significant differences. This is even true without taking into account culture-bound syndromes and trance and possession psychoses which occur outside of culturally authorized ritual settings. Those disorders by definition are found only or principally in non-Western societies. The epidemiological data, however, do not sustain the radical cultural relativist argument that mental disorders are incomparable in greatly different societies. The chief mental disorders are diagnosable worldwide; research is quite clear on this point. Thus, we are once again left with evidence of both cross-cultural universals and particularities, cross-cultural support for the dialectical view that "life requires both the determination of the environment and the physical body" (Kitaro 1970, p. 100).

Symptomatology

A salient international finding, often replicated as I have noted, is the marked predominance of somatic symptoms among depressed and anxious patients in non-Western societies, albeit these symptoms are also common in the West (Kleinman and Good, eds., 1985; Good and Kleinman 1985; Kirmayer 1984; H.B.M. Murphy 1982; Weiss and Kleinman in press).[5] Particular symptoms and symptom patterns differ across patients in different cultures. Because the literature relevant to symptomatology comes from studies of depression and anxiety disorders, I will focus principally on these conditions.

I have shown (1986) that headaches, dizziness, and lack of energy form a symptom cluster in ancient Chinese society and in contemporary Taiwan and China which is the core of neurasthenic illness behavior associated with mixed depressive and anxiety disorders. These symptoms have been culturally salient for centuries in Chinese society and still today carry considerable cultural meaning. Indeed, Chinese patients appear to selectively perceive, label, and communicate these symptoms out of the diffuse complaints of psychophysiological arousal and the multiform somatic effects of stress. The association of a culturally salient somatic language of complaints with depression and/or anxiety disorders has also been recorded for clinical samples in Saudi Arabia (Racy 1980), Iraq (Bazzoui 1970), Benin (Binitie 1975), Peru (Mezzich and Rabb 1980), India (Teja et al. 1971; Sethi et al. 1973), and Hong Kong (Cheung et al. 1981), and among depressed patients in many non-Western cultures (Marsella 1979).

Data from the WHO's cross-cultural study of depression in clinical research centers in Montreal, Teheran, Basel, Nagasaki, and Tokyo disclose both similarities and differences in symptomatology (Sartorius et al. 1983). Sadness, joylessness, anxiety, tension, lack of energy, decreased interest and concentration, and feelings of inadequacy and worthlessness were found in three-fourths to all of the depressed patients at each center. One-third had hypochondriacal ideas, and 40 percent had somatic complaints, obsessions, and phobias. More personality disorders were detected in Western centers, where concepts of such disorders may fit the Western diagnostic categories better, than in non-Western ones. Psychomotor agitation was more frequent in Teheran and symptoms of self-reproach higher in Europe. Marsella et al. (1985) reflect on their participation in this project and

HO comparison was not organized to pick up more center-
ms, and it didn't.

), working among the Ashanti in West Africa, in local heal-
ound that anxiety was commonly expressed as self-accusation
witchcraft. Studies in Nigerian society report that generalized
anxi... orders among Yoruba are associated with three clusters of primary symptoms—worries, dreams of witchcraft, and bodily complaints
(Collis, 1966; Anumonge 1970; Jegede 1978). Each of these takes a form
appropriate in Yoruba culture. Predominant worries expressed by patients
were those associated with procreation and maintenance of a large family.
Lambo (1962), himself a Yoruba psychiatrist, long ago noted the close correlation between "morbid fear of bewitchment" and "acute anxiety states
in Africa."

The combination of universal and culture-specific symptoms of depressive and anxiety disorders has been reported for Iranians (Good et
al. 1985), Chinese (Kleinman and Kleinman 1985), and American Indians
(Manson et al. 1985). Research on American Indians has shown that certain signs that might be taken as evidence of severe depression in other
groups are normative for members of this ethnic group, including "prolonged" mourning, "flat affect," auditory hallucinations of spirit beings,
and visual hallucinations of the recently dead (O'Nell, in press).

The research literature also points out that feelings of guilt are much
less commonly associated with depression in the non-Western world than
in the West. H.B.M. Murphy (1982) attributed guilt to the influence of
the Judeo-Christian heritage, including its effects on Islam. Melancholia,
the traditional term for depressive disorder in the West, acquired this
moral meaning from *acedia*, a religious expression of depression (Jackson
1985). But the literature purporting to demonstrate low frequency and severity of guilt in the Third World is flawed by the absence of consistent
definitions, operationalized criteria, and methods of assessment. This is
because many writers *assume* that guilt is a sign of higher levels of personality functioning—stronger egos, more intense superego development,
higher differentiation—on the basis of outmoded and unsubstantiated psychoanalytic and evolutionary schemes. Weiss and Kleinman (in press) note
that in spite of substantial findings of guilt in India (Venkoba Rao 1973;
Teja et al. 1971; Ansari 1969), discussions in the Indian literature minimize
its significance or interpret it as milder or of a different kind. For example,
Venkoba Rao (1973) distinguished karmic guilt (concerned with deeds in
a previous life) from present guilt. He felt that karmic guilt might actually
protect against the other type.

Sartorius et al. (1983) did not find major differences in guilt between
depressive patients in the West and Japan. Escobar and his co-workers
(1983), in keeping with H.B.M. Murphy's (1982) hypothesis, found Christian patients in Colombia to have the same degree of guilt in the course of

depression as found in depressed patients in North America. I (1986) discerned less guilt among depressives in China than is reported from the West, and noted that low self-esteem was also less common. I reviewed the work of Cheung and her colleagues (1981) in Hong Kong suggesting no major difference in guilt there and in the West, and wondered if her subjects are Christians or otherwise acculturated to Western values in that highly Westernized community. Since there are few studies that systematically look for other idioms of expressing guilt in the non-Western world, the finding of low preoccupation with guilt could be an artifact of reporting and of the research methodology.

For example, Field (1958) noted that the expression of guilt among her Ashanti informants occurred only in an idiom of witchcraft. Levy (1973), studying Tahitians, demonstrated in a subtle ethnographic and psychological study that shame and guilt were not discrete feelings, but intermixed. Lutz (1985), Rosaldo (1980), and other psychological anthropologists have studied individuals in small-scale preliterate societies whose concepts of self and emotions are radically different than in the West. These anthropologists repeatedly show that different meanings of guilt, sadness, and other emotions significantly influence the experience of those emotions (Lutz and White 1986). Guilt understood and experienced as existential suffering, or as loss of face, or as self-accusation of witchcraft is not the same emotional phenomenon. Thus, anthropologists hold that simple dichotomies between high and low levels of guilt or its presence and absence in very different societies distort a much more complex picture cross-culturally.

Suicide has also been said to be less common among depressed patients in the Third World (Headley, ed., 1983); it probably is, with some notable exceptions like Japan, less common in non-Western societies generally (La Fontaine 1975). But since most cases in developing societies probably go unrecorded, and since there is great variation across rural/urban, time, and ethnic boundaries, the cross-cultural epidemiology of suicide is anything but clear. Indeed, the low prevalence of suicide has been explained as the result of the alleged low level of guilt—a decidedly weak foundation.

I (1982) found less suicide among Chinese depressives in Hunan, but explained this finding by suggesting that somatization protects against this and other negative sequelae of a more intrapsychic, existential experience of depression. This explanation needs to be weighed against a history of salience of suicide in Chinese culture (Hsieh and Spence 1982). Mezzich and Raab (1980) report lower tendency toward suicide among depressed Peruvians than among matched North American depressives. They attribute this difference to strong teaching by the Catholic Church against suicide. Venkoba Rao points out several cultural factors in India that may protect against suicide. These include the emphasis on family obligations over individual rights, the legitimation of suicide, at least historically, under ritual conditions (*sati*), and the concept of *karma* (which would lead individuals to avoid suicide lest they be reborn in a less desirable state).

Attempted suicide in a number of Asian and Middle Eastern societies, as in North America, is higher among women than among men. But, unlike North America, completed suicides also appear to me more common among women in these societies (Headeley, ed., 1983). Reasons for suicide and means of carrying it out vary greatly, but there is significant evidence that relative powerlessness, absence of alternative means of communicating despair, traditional use of suicide as a sanctioned idiom of distress, and its place in cultural mythology make particular categories of women (generally the young but in certain cultures the elderly too) more likely, perhaps driven, to take this last alternative.

There is also evidence that social change contributes to fluctuating suicide rates. For example, suicide rates in various of the Pacific Island cultures are increasing rapidly as those societies experience the problems of modernization. Also a recent report from Sri Lanka reports that the suicide rate tripled between 1955 and 1974, when it was highest among the Tamil ethnic minority in the northeast (Kearney and Miller 1985). The authors explain the increase as the result of rapid population growth, increased competition for education and employment, and the breakdown of a stable society, placing great pressure especially on Tamils. It is unclear from their report whether these rates are associated with increased depression, or what has happened during the current era of civil war. Poverty, economic failure, and exam failure are other important social factors contributing to suicide around the globe. Much of the anthropological work on suicide has indicated that it may (and often does) occur in individuals without mental illness who are under great social pressure or for whom it is one of a very few culturally authorized expressions of severe distress (La Fontaine 1975).

The review of the findings of the WHO's cross-cultural comparison of schizophrenia, as noted earlier, also discloses important differences in the mode of onset and symptoms of schizophrenia. Barrett (in press), furthermore, offers evidence that the sense of a split or divided self that is so strongly associated with both professional and lay discourses on schizophrenia in the West may emerge as salient because of the Western conception of the person as a bounded individual self. Patients in the West report feeling a split in personality. This aspect of schizophrenia appears to be less central to the experience of the disorder in China and other non-Western societies. In those societies, the expression of a feeling of split personality is as uncommon as is the mythology of a self divided against itself.[6]

Thus, we can conclude that the symptomatology of mental disorders differs very substantially cross-culturally. For schizophrenia, major depressive disorder, and anxiety disorders there are also significant uniformities. If we lump together with these mental illnesses culture-bound disorders and trance-possession and other dissociative psychoses (occurring outside ritually prescribed settings), then the variation in the symptoms of mental illness is much greater. Thus, the research literature on symptomatology points to the same pattern of cross-cultural findings as do the other aspects of mental illness we have reviewed: there are certain significant similarities and many very significant differences.[7]

Illness Behavior

Few researchers have actually compared the illness behavior—i.e., meaningful experience of symptoms and patterns of coping and help seeking—of appropriately matched samples of depressed or anxious patients in different societies. Research does disclose, however, greatly different patterns of help seeking for mental illness in different societies and ethnic groups (Lin et al. 1978; Lin, Kleinman and Lin 1982). These studies find, for example, that North American Indian, Asian, and Caucasian ethnic patients follow distinctive pathways to the mental health center, arrive there at very different points in the course of illness, and experience greatly divergent types of involvement of their family members. Response to psychiatric treatment also differs. Lin et al. (1986) review the literature demonstrating distinctive pharmacokinetic and pharmacodynamic responses to tricyclic antidepressants among East Asian and Caucasian groups, disclosing different physiological responses to treatment in these ethnic groups. That is to say, biology-culture interactions are important in treatment, and are probably also significant in perception of symptoms (cf. Hoosain 1986).

Perhaps the best way to get at cultural influences on illness perception and experience in mental illnesses like depressive and anxiety disorders is to analyze those culture-bound syndromes that bear a family resemblance to these disorders, because certain of these syndromes have been described in considerable detail. Manson et al. (1985) disclose that among Hopi one culture-specific syndrome overlaps extensively with depressive symptomatology, whereas several others that appear to overlap actually are distinctive. Johnson and Johnson (1965) discovered among the Dakota Sioux a syndrome called *towatl ye sni* (or "totally discouraged"). This syndrome cut across various Western categories of psychopathology, but struck the authors as especially close to depression. Yet the beliefs and behaviors labeled *towatl ye sni* were also strongly culturally shaped and included feelings of deprivation, the experience of one's thoughts traveling to the dwelling place of dead relatives, an orientation to the past as the best time, willing death to become nearer to the dead, and preoccupations with ghosts and spirits.

Prince and Tcheng-Laroche (1987) show that *taijinkyofusho* among Japanese can be glossed as a phobia of interpersonal relations but is different from DSM-III social phobia inasmuch as patients feel guilty about embarrassing others with their behavior (e.g., blushing, unpleasant body odor, stuttering) rather than fearful of others' criticisms. In *taijinkyofusho* the emphasis is on the fear of discomfiting others through their sense of shame, a fear thoroughly in concert with Japanese cultural sensibilities but quite foreign to North American fears. This experience suggests that psychiatric classifications of phobias are insufficient as presently cast to model a major illness experience in Japanese society. While similarities have been found between agoraphobia and one type of neurasthenia in Japan, *shinkeishitsu* associated with obsessions and phobias, there are also divergences. Agoraphobia in North America is found predominantly in women, *shinkeishitsu* in men. Western sufferers are afraid of being alone in public; Japanese patients avoid contact with others (least with intimates or strangers, most with acquaintances). The illness behavior of the Japanese is best described as "anthropophobic."

Littlewood and Lipsedge (1987) argue that anorexia nervosa might be regarded as a culture-specific illness behavior in the West, at times associated with personality disorder, at other times part of a constellation of psychiatric depression with somatic delusions. These British psychiatrists point out anorexia nervosa is not highly prevalent outside the West, with the exception of the educated class of industrialized societies like Japan who have been strongly influenced by Western aesthetic standards which value extreme slimness and which view strict dieting as an emblem of moral discipline. The historian Caroline Walker Bynum (in press), who traces the lineaments of anorexia to various Christian saints, concludes:

> The cultures within which female non-eating occurs and achieves significance as a form of sanctity or empowerment are all cultures which, on the one hand, associate the female with body and sexuality and, on the other, expect females to suffer and to serve (especially to offer food to) others.

Anorectic women in medieval Italy and modern Portugal participate, she avers, not in behavior whose cause is physiological, but in cultures which share similar perceptions of women's roles and symbolism of being female. Historical analysis does not lend support, furthermore, to psychodynamic interpretations of the nature of mother-daughter conflict or patriarchal control as the basis for anorectic behavior. The "starving disease" epidemic of our time, she shows, is also more than the fight among a male-dominated culture and a resisting female subculture for control of the bodies of adolescent girls that feminist psychologists have made it out to be. The symbolic meaning in modern Portuguese peasant society and medieval Italy of noneating as purity through suffering that brings women, who are otherwise symbolically polluting, closer to God, Bynum regards as the most availing explanation for anorexia in those societies. The noneating living, like the consecrated incorrupt dead, "symbolize restraint or purity that harnesses and channels, but does not destroy, fertility" (see also Bell

1985; Pina-Cabral 1986). Brian Turner (1985, pp. 180–201), a sociologist who has canvassed the social historical significance of bodily practices in the West, links the cultural analysis of anorexia with the political and economic forces in contemporary capitalism's consumer society to show that this is a disorder whose sign—slimness—is promoted by food and drug and other industries for which this bodily product of hedonism and narcissism holds powerful commercial significance.

What can be generalized from these and many, many other accounts is that illness behavior is always strongly shaped by culture even when the associated disease processes can be diagnosed with an international nosology. Whatever the causes of anorexia, which are likely to be multiple and interactive, the experience of anorexia and other chronic disorders is inseparable from their cultural context.

Course and Outcome

A final aspect of illness behavior, but one deserving special attention, is course and outcome of disorder. Here the literature is particularly murky. The example of better outcome for schizophrenia in less developed societies is a beam of clear light. One of the more interesting (and better-supported) hypotheses to explain this finding is Waxler's (1977) theory that where schizophrenia is popularly viewed as an acute problem and patients suffering from it are accordingly expected to recover just like those who suffer from other acute disorders, there the cultural message is reinforced by familial and community responses to the patient that encourage normalization and discourage acceptance of a disabled role. In this view, chronicity is in large measure the result of social messages and interpersonal reactions to the patient that impede the patient's sense of self-control and undermine his optimism and its psychophysiological effects. Other factors such as the economics of disability, the investment of certain mental health programs in maintaining patients in long-term patient roles, and the very high demands that industrialized societies make on former patients in the absence of effective supports have also been implicated as obstacles to better outcome from schizophrenia (Lin and Kleinman in press; Warner 1985; Estroff 1981; Waxler 1977). The medical profession may inadvertently abet these forces, since in North American and Western European society its members have been trained to treat schizophrenic patients with the expectation that there is little that can be done to help them recover from a disorder that until recently was regarded as progressively disabling. In fact, more recent long-term research shows that even in the West, the course of many schizophrenic patients is much more hopeful than the professional stereotype (see Bleuler 1978; Harding et al. 1987; Alanen et al. 1986).

If we take suicide as an outcome, then somatized illness experience in major depressive disorder in the Third World would have a better outcome than psychologized depression in the West, inasmuch as there is less suicide among the former group. But given what has already been said about the relationship of guilt and low self-esteem to depression, and taking into account the tendency toward lower suicide rates generally in much of the nonindustrialized world, it is difficult to be certain if somatization per se protects against suicide. However, because of the findings for schizophrenia in developing societies, it is important that research be undertaken to compare the course of depressive and anxiety disorders in Western and non-Western societies. A leading hypothesis should be that somatized depression may have an easier course and better outcome than psychologized depression, owing to less morbid preoccupation with, and negative expectation in, the personal experience of the illness.

Overall, then, chronicity and disability may be at least partially separable from physiological disease processes and their causes. Just as there is no one-to-one correlation of symptom to pathology, there are a variety of courses for the same disorder. The meanings of the illness experience and the social context of the sick person together with his biography also shape these outcomes (Osterweis et al., eds., 1987). It is unlikely that all or even most non-Western settings encourage processes of adaptation and rehabilitation, but clearly contemporary industrialized societies place certain categories of the sick under constraints that foster chronicity and disability. This is a topic that is likely to receive much greater attention in future cross-cultural research.

Illness Beliefs

In 1976, in a provocative article aimed at disputing the claims of labeling theorists that mental illness was influenced by the type of label and societal response it elicited, J. Murphy claimed that major psychiatric disorder— i.e., insanity—is similarly identified and labeled cross-culturally. Subsequently, Westermeyer and Wintrob (1979) reviewed some of the literature on folk models of mental illness in a number of societies and came to the conclusion that all the societies in their review possessed a notion of madness (cf. White 1982 for a corresponding view). In a later paper, Murphy (1982:70) put the case this way:

> . . . there seems to be little that is distinctively cultural in the attitudes and actions directed toward the mentally ill. . . . There is apparently a common range of possible responses to the mentally ill person, and the portion of the range brought to bear regarding a particular person is determined more by the nature of his or her behavior than by a preexisting cultural set to respond in a uniform way to whatever is labelled mental illness.

On the other hand, ethnographic studies demonstrate convincingly that concepts of emotions, self and body, and general illness categories differ so significantly in different cultures that it can be said that each culture's beliefs about normal and abnormal behavior are distinctive (cf. Good 1977; Rosaldo 1980; Kleinman and Good, eds., 1985; Lutz and White 1986; Marsella et al. 1985; G. Lewis 1975; Janzen 1978; and Leslie, ed., 1976, to list only a few examples). Townsend (1978), for example, showed that even in the West the beliefs of Germans and North Americans about major mental disorder were fundamentally divergent and strongly influenced the views of mental health professionals in each of the societies to such an extent that German patients and psychiatrists held more similar views than did German and North American psychiatrists.

My interpretation of this controversy follows the line of reasoning that led me to argue for a culture-biology dialectic in the understanding of disorder. Certain disorders such as florid psychosis—i.e., madness—appear to be significantly constrained by shared psychobiological processes so that their form bears a resemblance in different societies. At the same time there are significant differences in the content of symptoms and mode of their expression owing to cultural context. The uniform psychobiology of the disease process would seem to delimit the categories of psychosis so that there is rough (but by no means complete) agreement worldwide on what behaviors constitute madness—hallucinations, delusions, inability to test reality, highly inappropriate and at times violent behavior, etc.—though the imputed causes are greatly different.

Even for the category madness, however, there are important cross-cultural differences in the details: the most salient symptoms, the level of symptom frequency or intensity that leads to the label, the nature and degree of stigma, and so forth. Jenkins (in press) shows, for example, that Mexican-American families frequently identify the problem of their schizophrenic members as *nervios* ("nerves"), which is less stigmatizing than the use of a language of madness, is associated with lower levels of negative expressed emotion, and "may differentially allow for the continued incorporation of the ill person within social groups." T. Y. Lin and M. C. Lin (1982) indicate that the stigma associated with categorizing individuals as mad in Chinese culture is more severe than that in the West, since the stigma attaches not just to the afflicted member but to the family as a whole. Hence for the most severe psychiatric disorder there is evidence of both uniformity and difference across different cultures. For other mental illnesses the picture is not at all the same. Whether a problem is called a mental illness, what characteristics lead to that description, the full range of beliefs about cause, onset of symptoms at a particular time, reason for vulnerability, pathophysiology, expected course, and appropriate treatment vary so greatly that the presumption that culture always particularizes receives overwhelming confirmation. The most diverse conceptualizations are drawn on to explain emotional problems such as depression or anxiety and behaviors such as use of alcohol and drugs and other forms of deviance. Cultures may have no label for depression as a category or may conceive of sadness in ways that make no sense in Western society (Rosaldo 1980; Schieffelin 1985). The values attached to these categories and the actions they authorize also are greatly distinctive. Qat—an addictive drug—is in Yemen used by almost the entire male population—not to use it would be regarded as social deviance (Weir 1980; Kennedy 1987). Lutz (1985) goes so far as to reason from this wealth of diversity among indigenous belief systems that professional psychological categories too are best viewed as one kind of ethnopsychology.

Psychophysiological Experiences

One of the most provocative findings in cross-cultural research must be the evidence that trance and possession states are ubiquitous in non-Western societies and were so in the West prior to the modern age.[8] Among certain traditionally oriented subgroups in North America and Europe, they persist as a lively aspect of alternative consciousness. Viewed in this manner, only the modern, secular West seems to have blocked individuals' access to these otherwise pan-human dimensions of the self. Perhaps this transformation can be understood via T. S. Eliot's observation that the individual in the modern West suffers from a "dissociation of sensibility" which, as the noted psychoanalytic revisionist Charles Rycroft (1986) puts it, "compels him to change his stance perpetually and to shift uneasily from participating emotionally in life and adapting the pose he is above and outside the system which he is observing objectively." This split in consciousness, which the German phenomenologist Plessner (1970) referred to as the experience of simultaneously being a body and having a body, we associate with the rise of a discursive, metatheoretical "modernist" orientation to the self that is secular, self-reflexive, and ironic. This acquired consciousness interferes with total absorption in lived experience, which is the essence of the highly focused state of attention characteristic of trance. It also renders less available the hysterical state of overt, dramatic bodily response to life shocks. The rationalizing powers of modern secular Western society have either created or intensified a metaself—a critical observer who watches and comments on experience. The self is alienated from unreflected, unmediated experience. By internalizing a critical observer, the self is rendered inaccessible to possession by gods or ghosts; it cannot faint from fright or become paralyzed by humiliation; it loses the literalness of bodily metaphors of the most intimate personal distress, accepting in their place a psychological metalanguage that has the appearance of immediacy but in fact distances felt experience; and the self becomes vulnerable to forms of pathology (like borderline and narcissistic personality disorders) that appear culture-bound to the West.

Indeed, the self as we come to know and experience it is a "construction" of modern culture. That modern construction has deepened discursive layers of experience (e.g., the cognitive competence to differentiate dysphoria into distinctive states of depression and anxiety and the linguistic competence to use emotional talk) while paradoxically making more difficult to grasp and communicate poetic, moral, and spiritual layers of the felt flow of living. Trance and posesssion are not, as some psychologists and psychiatrists aver, "primitive" forms of pathology. Rather they are ways of experiencing and articulating the body/self in nondualistic, archaic tropes. Here category transforms experience. When they occur in culturally authorized ritual and group settings, they are normative and normal. When they occur outside these settings, they are best regarded as culturally shaped, psychobiologically based dissociative processes in which different layers of experience (or ways of communicating experience) are split off into indwelling icons (or semiotic systems) of gods, ghosts, or ancestors. When associated with floridly psychotic behavior, these processes are likely to be maladaptive. Here experience transforms category. The affected person does not just get labeled, but becomes possessed.

What is it in the structure of certain cultures that fosters the embodied experience of particular categories? Are trance among peasants in India and possession among rural dwellers in Bali indwelling metaphors shaping the same core experiences as existential angst expresses among the upper middle class in Manhattan? Or do cultural category and idiom create felt experience? Are somatization and psychologization yet another aspect of this psychocultural transformation? Can personalities be reproduced, as Lasch (1979) argues they can, so as to replicate in motivation and coping style the key tensions in society? For example, do the bottomless desire and empty emotional superficiality of borderline personality reproduce on the individual plane the cultural requirements of capitalism? Is Type A personality as culturally adaptive as it is psychobiologically dysfunctional? That is to say, is it too an example of the cultural reproduction of personality? Or do these salient personality pathologies arise from a genetic basis as has recently been claimed? (Baron et al. 1985; Kendler et al. 1984; Torgerson 1984). Few definitive answers are available, but enough is know to generate provocative questions in the borderland between psychology and culture.

The chief conclusion of this review is that the reciprocal influence between cultural category and personal experience (which itself is the result of interaction between norms, relationships, and the body-self) both proliferates cross-cultural differences in mental illness and constrains the type and degree of divergence. A reading of one side of the spectrum or the other in isolation is unavailing and tendentious; it is blind to that which is cross-cultural research's greatest lesson: categories are embodied in persons, experiences are taken up (and transformed) within cultures' meaning systems.

Chapter 4

Do Social Relations and Cultural Meanings Contribute to the Onset and Course of Mental Illness?

————————◆————————

. . . human misery has awakened, stood before you, and today demands its
proper place.

Jean Jaurès, 1897,
cited in J.D. Bredin, *The Affair*

There is, then, a critical difference between the way we estimate the
"heritability" of a trait and the way we usually interpret such estimates. Since
there is no practical method for separating the physical and social effects of
genes, heritability estimates include both. This means that heritability estimates
set a lower bound on the explanatory power of the environment, not an upper
bound. If genetic variation explains 60 percent of the variation in IQ scores,
environmental variation must *explain the remaining 40 percent, but it* may
explain as much as 100 percent. If, for example, genes affected IQ scores solely
by affecting children's appearance or behavior, and if their appearance or
behavior then affected the way they were treated at home or at school,
everything genes explained would also be explicable by environmental factors.

Christopher Jencks,
Genes and Crime

There are really three questions to consider. The first is *whether* social
forces contribute to the onset and course of mental illness and therefore
do, or can, play a role in its prevention. The evidence is so overwhelmingly
in favor of a significant contribution of the social environment to the origin
and exacerbation of mental disorders that we will be able to answer this

question quickly. The second question—*how* do social relations and cultural meanings exert such an effect?—is a much more complicated issue, but we can outline a general answer, even if the technical details require more research before they can be precisely described. The third question is, what implications do, or should, the answers to the first two questions hold for psychiatrists?

Let us first marshal the pertinent sources of information to answer the initial question. Then we can critique the dominant concept and research methodology in studies of the relationship of social environment to mental illness—namely, the "stress, social support, illness onset" model. Our critique will provide the point of departure for a different paradigm of the way the social environment contributes to mental illness. Following that, we will be in a position to examine obstacles to the effective use of information on the social contribution to the causes of mental illness by the psychiatric profession and to its application in preventive programs. Having gone so far, we are obliged to suggest how the profession might usefully respond to these findings. That question I will explicitly address in the final two chapters.

Political Economy And Mental Illness

The evidence for an influence of the social world on mental illness comes from a variety of studies at different levels of analysis. Economists have shown that the state of the economy in North American society over the past 100 years or so is a useful predictor of rates of hospital admissions for mental illness and of suicides (Brenner 1981). The poor are more than twice as likely as others to report themselves in poor health (Robert Wood Johnson Foundation 1987, p. 5). Most mental disorders have their highest prevalence rate in the lowest socioeconomic class.[1] And in North American society, members of black and Hispanic minority ethnic groups, who are overrepresented in the lowest socioeconomic class, are also at higher risk for such disorders, though there are major intraethnic differences (Angel and Thoits 1987; Karno et al. 1987; Canino et al. 1987; Moscicki et al. 1987). Furthermore, the 1986 National Access Survey shows it is precisely these groups whose access to care has decreased (Robert Wood Johnson Foundation 1987).

Warner (1985) has analyzed the prevalence and outcome of schizophrenia in relation to the political economy. His analysis, as I mentioned in the preceding chapter, discloses the close relationship between illness onset, treatment outcome, and the vicissitudes of employment, on the one hand, and the economic situation, on the other. At this point it is worth examining his argument in detail, since it is the most impressive analysis of this subject. Warner adverts to the evidence that first-time admissions

to the hospital increase in times of high unemployment, and that the prevalence of schizophrenia seems to be lower in those parts of the nonindustrialized world where wage labor has not developed and higher in those sections of the industrial world where there is high unemployment. Where
wage labor exists in developing societies, those classes most negatively affected by labor conditions and unemployment appear to be at greater risk
for schizophrenia. The incidence of schizophrenia among immigrants is
higher than in their country of origin if they encounter "harsher labor conditions in their new country." Warner argues from the available evidence
that schizophrenia is more common in the sex that faces the harshest labor-
market conditions and that the age at which this severe mental illness has
its onset is determined by the age at which men and women enter the labor
market. Drawing on historical sources, he supports the contention that the
dramatic increase in wage labor during the eighteenth and nineteenth centuries correlated with a rise in the occurrence of schizophrenia in the industrialized West.

Warner's analysis of the outcome of schizophrenia builds on the following pieces of evidence: spending on psychiatric hospital care increases during times of economic depression; during the Great Depression there was
a decreased rate of recovery from schizophrenia because of the effect of
economic stress and unemployment on patients in the community; many of
the negative symptoms of chronic schizophrenia—e.g., depression, apathy,
irritability, negativity, emotional overdependence, social withdrawal, isolation, loneliness, and loss of self-esteem, loss of identity, and loss of a sense
of time—are similar to what have been described as the sequelae of long-
term unemployment. Warner indicates too that rehabilitation efforts for
the chronic mentally ill go up and down with the business cycle and that
schizophrenics who are more readily employed (women, higher-class patients) have a better outcome, and he marshals what data are available
to build the case that outcome for schizophrenia may be better in full-
employment societies than in other industrialized societies that tolerate
(and even depend on) a high rate of "natural" unemployment. Warner
uses the WHO data and those of Murphy and Raman (1971) and
Waxler (1979), which show better outcome of schizophrenia in patients in
developing societies, to support his contention that the modern system of
wage labor is as much the culprit as is unemployment per se.* Warner also
believes chronic drug therapy may actually worsen the long-term course

---

*Better outcome from schizophrenia in the less socially developed societies may not have
anything to do with wage labor. That is only one hypothesis to explain this finding. As I noted
in Chapter 3, there are other explanations for differential outcome, such as different levels of
social isolation and social support in developing and developed societies; major differences in
the structure and functioning of families; different expectations of chronicity and disability;
variation in stigma; and differential survival of vulnerable individuals (see Lin and Kleinman
1987).*

of schizophrenia by amplifying withdrawal symptoms in good-prognosis patients and contributing to the very biological problems in the brain that many researchers believe underwrite the disorder. Thus, the so-called "negative" symptoms of shizophrenia—e.g., inertia and apathy—may be results of chronic drug therapy (see also Alanen et al. 1986).

Some of the inferences Warner draws between the political economy and mental illness, such as his argument linking the so-called absence of wage labor and supposedly lower rates of schizophrenia in non-Western societies, are controversial. Others are interpretive leaps from a fairly limited data base. The chief conclusions about the effect of the political economy on mental illness are, on the other hand, well supported. Nor are these the only pertinent findings that demonstrate the contribution of the social environment to mental illness. Hugh Freeman (1984), a senior British psychiatrist and editor of the prestigious *British Journal of Psychiatry*, in a comprehensive survey of the scientific study of mental health and the environment, adduces additional potential wellsprings of mental ill health, for which the research evidence is at least suggestive, including crowding, other aspects of the urban environment such as information overload, noise, poor housing, population mobility, and violence, and social isolation, social disintegration, and the topic to which I will now turn, social change.

Social Change and Other Social Contributions to Mental Illness

As noted earlier, major social change in Taiwan from the late 1940s to the middle 1960s was associated with a very large increase in the rates of neurotic disorders (Lin et al. 1969). Yeh et al. (1987) present evidence that this correlation persists and even intensifies in the 1970s and 80s. Leighton and his coworkers (1963) demonstrated that social breakdown in communities correlates with increased rates of mental distress.[2] Alcoholism and drug abuse and suicide become major mental health risks during periods of rapid modernization of traditionally oriented populations—e.g., North American Indians, Alaskan Natives, and South Pacific, New Guinean, and East Asian populations (Kraus and Bufler 1979; Shore and Manson 1983; Beiser 1985; Rubinstein 1985; Lin, Kleinman and Lin 1982). Uprooting and forced acculturation among refugees, immigrants, and migrants have repeatedly been shown to create increased rates of mental illnesses. For example, Southeast Asian "boat people" who have resettled in North America experience high rates of depression, anxiety, and psychophysiological disturbances (Beiser and Fleming 1986). Some social problems are so common among particular minority populations—e.g., "antisocial personality" among inner-city black youth in the United States, "family pathology" among urban slum dwellers in Egypt and in many other areas of the world—as to be almost modal (Wikan 1980). These can be shown to represent long-term responses to historical forces that create an underclass in society. Worldwide, women in most studies bear higher rates of mental illness than men, and research points to the importance of their relative powerlessness (Weissman and Klerman 1977; Brown and Harris 1978). For example, working-class and middle-income women under the greatest pressure at home, without jobs outside the home, and who have the least social support from spouse and friends are at greater risk to succumb to clinical depression (Brown and Harris 1978). As that powerlessness and deprivation worsens, so too will the burden of mental illness. Extreme conditions, such as the Holocaust, the Cambodian genocide, the Vietnam War, and the Cultural Revolution in China, also increase the long-term burden of mental distress and disorder (Dimsdale, ed., 1980; Lifton 1983, 1986; Thurston 1987; Eisenbruch 1986).

Even among sufferers from that mental disorder which is believed by many to carry the greatest degree of biological loading—schizophrenia—family and cultural forces (described in the preceding chapter) influence onset, course, and outcome (Brown et al. 1962; Brown, Birley, and Wing 1972; Vaughn and Leff 1976; Day et al. 1987; Waxler 1979). Family pathology correlates with a wide range of psychiatric disturbance (Reiss 1981; Minuchin et al. 1978; McGoldrick et al., eds., 1982). I do not have the space to review the many studies of mental health and work, but the data argue for a significant role of unemployment, problematic work relationships, and stressful work conditions in the development of mental health problems (e.g., Brenner 1987; Brenner and Levi 1987; Frese and Mohr 1987; Levi 1984; Rose, Hurst, and Herd 1979; Joelson and Wahlquist 1987). Life event changes perceived as stressful—bereavement, divorce, other key losses and threats—have been repeatedly shown to precede the onset of mental illness, whereas adequate social support and coping resources have been found to protect individuals from these problems (Berkman 1981; Eisenberg 1980; Dohrenwend and Dohrenwend 1974; Horowitz 1976; Paykel et al. 1969; Henderson 1981, 1982; Henderson and Moran 1983; Henderson et al. 1986; N. Lin et al. 1979, 1986; Rutter 1986). For example, death of a spouse, parent or child significantly increases the risk for developing clinical depression and drug and alcohol abuse one year later (Clayton 1974, 1979, 1982). Men below the age of 75 in North America, furthermore, have been shown to experience greater mortality after bereavement when compared to nonbereaved controls (Osterweis et al. 1984). Those who remarried reduced this risk. Mechanic (1986), reviewing the major social science findings, demonstrates that social class, the economy, historical forces influencing the movement of one's birth cohort through the life course, and social institutions are the chief determinants of health and mental well-being.

Social policies also contribute to the problem. The findings of pertinent research on comprehensive community care for the chronically mentally ill consistently demonstrate that this can be an effective alternative to inpatient psychiatric treatment for many of these individuals (Brown et al. 1981; Liberman and Phipps 1984). But deinstitutionalization of the chronically mentally ill in the United States has not been accompanied by the provision of the necessary resources to develop such community programs. Rather the mentally ill have simply been dumped onto the street to reduce the cost of inpatient programs and to give the impression of concern with their civil rights. Poor, without jobs, isolated, homeless, victimized, the deinstitutionalized mentally ill have had their income maintenance benefits cut by the Social Security Administration in the absence of effective rehabilitation programs. The result is that they are incarcerated in jails or nursing homes, subject to revolving-door recidivism in mental hospitals, and placed in conditions of utter misery that cannot but worsen the course of disease just as they render inhuman the experience of illness (Estroff 1981, pp. 258–276). Perhaps nothing so poignantly illustrates the vicious cycles in which the unrelieved social consequences of severe mental illness feed back to become the social antecedents of relapse, rehospitalization, and disability.

The reader must not overinterpret what I am concluding. There is no evidence that social factors are the sole determinant of mental disorders. Among individuals in those social groups that experience the most severe social pressures with the least resources to protect them, many experience distress, but most do not develop a mental disorder (Rutter 1986). Causation of mental disease is such a complex interaction between biological and psychological and social sources of vulnerability to the peril of precipitating events—one type of vulnerability intensified by the others not as separable risk factors but as a systematically interrelated web of susceptibility— that the term causation itself can be misleading. I prefer, therefore, to speak of social influences that place particular categories of persons at great risk for the onset of mental disorder or that contribute to the worsening of the course of disorder. In the onset of most episodes of mental disorder, one simply cannot say "this alone was the cause."

Prevention and Human Misery

It seems difficult, then, to argue against the conclusion that the social environment significantly influences the onset and course of mental disorder. However, data on prevention, based on this nexus of influence, are only beginning to become available. Bereavement counseling and self-help groups appear to ameliorate the long-term negative effects of bereavement in at-risk populations, though the studies supporting this finding are plagued by technical problems (Osterweis et al. 1984). It has been difficult to demonstrate conclusively that social interventions significantly reduce the burdens of mental health problems among high-risk American Indian and other minority groups. But the kinds of preventive measures introduced in such studies usually are quite minimal when compared to the magnitude of social problems (Eisenberg 1987; Manson, ed., 1982; McDermott et al. 1972). It is reasonable to expect that where substantial social interventions are propagated together with effective therapeutic modalities, prevention will have a greater likelihood of success; and there is early evidence in favor of this hypothesis (Kunitz 1983; Manson, ed., 1982; Frese 1987). Several studies suggest that when schizophrenic patients and their support networks receive adequate social resources (income, jobs, rehabilitation training, counseling) to cope with chronicity, rehospitalization and disability can be significantly reduced (Estroff, 1981, p. 259). Chronic illness behavior can be limited and its more negative consequences controlled through tertiary prevention, such as intervention in the family to reduce negative expressed emotion and improve family functioning (Leff et al. 1982; Hogarty and Goldberg 1973; Falloon et al. 1982).

The way I have presented these data implies that mental health problems are discrete from other kinds of misfortune. But, in fact, the case has been presented the other way round. Depression and anxiety disorders resulting from social causes can be reconceived not as discrete diseases, but rather as nonspecific bodily (psychobiological) forms of human distress (Antonovsky 1979; Cacioppo and Petty, eds., 1983; Shacter and Singer 1962). Why distinguish these problems simply because at times they exhibit distinctive forms of symptom presentation, when they share the same social origins? Demoralization and despair owing to severe family, work, or economic problems trigger syndromes of distress that have biological as well as psychological correlates. These correlates are often labeled psychiatric disorder, but they have been reconceived by social scientists as the psychobiological sequelae of social pathology and human misery generally. Even when genetic predisposition and neurobiological vulnerability convert the experiential effect of social pressures here into depressive disorder, there into panic disorder, the sociosomatic transduction can be with greater parsimony configured as simply social distress. Seen from this wider perspective, what is important is not so much the diverging form of the psychobiological response as the similar social antecedents.

In clinical and epidemiological research up until the 1960s, psychiatrists, strongly influenced by psychoanalytic thinking, looked upon neuroses—hysteria, depressive disorder, anxiety disorders—more as a spectrum of psychophysiological distress than as discrete disorders. The term "psychoneurosis" was often used as a diagnosis for a wide variety of disturbances. The concept of reaction to stress, popularized by the influential Johns Hopkins psychiatrist Adolph Meyer, was integral to this formulation (see Rutter 1986). Later, with the introduction of allegedly specific treatments for individual conditions—depression, panic, phobias, and so forth—the current viewpoint that neuroses are a group of separate disease states became ascendant. The product of this disease-specific viewpoint is DSM-III, which has replaced the rubric "neurosis" with clusters of discrete disorders. Each cluster originates from inclusion and exclusion criteria that enable the clinician to diagnose overlapping conditions as independent diseases; e.g., the anxiety disorders cluster specifies the criteria to distinguish generalized anxiety disorder, panic disorder, obsessive-compulsive disorders, agoraphobia, social phobia, and simple phobia. The idea is that each has a distinctive psychobiology, cause, course, and treatment response.

Many data do not fit well into this formulation. First, treatment specificity is not nearly as clear-cut as originally claimed. Antidepressants can be used to treat certain anxiety disorders; certain "anxiolytics" have an effect against depression. Behavioral and other psychotherapies work with almost all the neuroses (Beck 1976; Klein et al. 1983). Second, for all the recent research interest in neurotic conditions, there is little evidence that their causes are distinctive (Carr and Vitaliano 1985; Coyne 1976; Seligman 1975). Even the biological concomitants disclose great overlap. The hormonal changes characteristic of clinical depression have not been found to be pathognomonic. Panic disorder has been shown to have a unique brain focus of asymmetric cerebral blood flow (Reiman et al. 1984)—a study yet to be replicated. Otherwise, autonomic nervous system and limbic system changes appear to be nonspecific in depression and anxiety. Moreover, anxiety often accompanies depression, so that the two are not easily separable. One cannot say with confidence which is primary. It might be more rational to think of a continuum of psychobiological responses from "pure" anxiety to "pure" depression, with most cases falling in between. Finally, these discrepant findings can be explained by an alternative theory, which can be described as follows.

Psychological and biological vulnerability of the person combines with local social pressures to create syndromes of distress embodying neuroendocrine, autonomic, cardiovascular, gastrointestinal, and limbic system responses. Such responses constitute a spectrum of affective, anxiety, and somatic complaints. Cultural norms reciprocally interact with biological processes to pattern these body/self experiences so that different archetypes of distress are predominant in different social groups, such as neurasthenia in contemporary China, *fatigué* in France, chronic pain in North America, *nervios* in Latin America, and so on. Interpersonal and intrapsychic influences also shape the psychobiology of the neurotic response (Coyne 1976), which is perhaps more accurately described by the sociological concept of illness behavior (Mechanic, ed. 1982). That is to say, the "disease" in neurotic disorder is the nonspecific psychobiological changes of distress, demoralization, and fear (Tyrer 1986). The illness behavior, elaborated and interpreted variously in different cultures, may be anorexia, dysthymia, agoraphobia, *taijinkyofusho*, panic disorder, or the latest fad, chronic viral syndromes (Knox 1987; Berris 1986; Hofstadter 1987).

From this social viewpoint, the neuroses represent the medicalization of socially caused psychophysiological syndromes of human misery. Cross-cultural research presents significant evidence in favor of this hypothesis (Kleinman and Good, eds., 1985; Murphy 1982; Beiser and Fleming 1986). For example, Southeast Asian refugees in Canada respond to the serious stress of acculturation with psychophysiological syndromes of demoralization and fear that include various packages of discrete symptoms of anxiety, depression, and physical complaints, e.g., abdominal discomfort or so-called Southeast Asian belly (Beiser 1985). Many share these nonspecific complaints, but each of the packages differs somewhat. The diagnostic categories of the clinical researcher and the particular vulnerabilities of the person and the group "determine" which of these packages are elaborated and interpreted as major depressive disorder and which as panic disorder. From this social perspective, neuroses are not diseases, but socially induced behavioral manifestations of distress (Abramson et al. 1978; Bandura 1977; Coyne et al. 1981; Carr and Vitaliano 1985).

Human misery of all kinds is greater among the poor, the oppressed, the helpless. Why single out psychiatric disorder? The evidence for the autonomy of many psychiatric problems remains equivocal. Dysthymia will strike many as only a technical euphemism for unhappiness, hysterical personality disorder as a medical shorthand for uncooperation from aggressive or attention-seeking female patients, who might regard both the term and the doctors who use it as paternalistic and unempathetic (Thompson and Goldberg 1987). Indeed, most disorders—including a wide range of medical disorders—have their highest prevalence rate among the poor and disadvantaged (Black 1980). In this sense, they can also be viewed as socially caused forms of human misery, which physicians euphemistically gloss as "life problems." Life problems make up between one-third and two-thirds of the problems in medical practice (Katon et al. 1982). There is little doubt that major social change which leads to improved housing, better diet, control of water and sewage, higher levels of education, and employment is the chief source of improved health status, mortality rates, and disease statistics, though public health and health care technologies also make a contribution (McKeown 1976a, 1976b; Eisenberg 1984; Mechanic 1982; Navarro 1986). Rethinking medicine from the vantage point of these findings leads to the proposition that much of ill health is but one domain of human misery, and that the lion's share of that misery takes its origin from sociopolitical, socioeconomic, and sociopsychological affairs.

Of course, the specificity and nonspecificity models can be made to be complementary, as wave and particle theories are in physics. We can understand the tragic experience of Mrs. Lin Xiling, in Chapter 1, as a syndrome of profound distress caused by serious losses and a destructive family circle, or as a more discrete psychiatric disorder, depression, for which a specifically effective treatment is available, or as the elaboration of the former into the latter under the influence of her personal experience and our cultural and professional categories.

Effective preventive efforts require better knowledge of *how* social and cultural problems conduce to mental disorder. That is this chapter's second and more difficult question.

George Brown and his colleague Terril Harris (1978) have formulated an influential model of how vulnerability factors interact with precipitating events to create depression. Their model builds, at least implicitly, upon the theory of the American psychologist Seligman (1975; cf. Abrahamson et al. 1978), who reasons from studies of animals and humans that depression results from learned helplessness. Brown and Harris identify biological, psychological, and social factors that make the person vulnerable to the effect of serious stressful life events, like significant losses which generalize from situational feelings of specific hopelessness to overall pessimism and despair. This process of generalizing hopelessness transforms social pressures into psychological problems; hence, a vulnerable young working-class woman, deserted by her own mother when a child and sexually abused by her father, responds to loss of job and a physically abusive alcoholic husband with grieving, guilt, a feeling of worthlessness, and thoughts of suicide which then turn into a habitual behavioral pattern. Those psychological reactions, in turn, trigger or intensify the biology of clinical depression. Brown's hypothesis directs prevention to more precise interventions to treat or prevent depressive disorder—job training and placement, marital counseling, assistance with child care and homemaking, referral to appropriate social agencies, individual and group psychotherapy, etc.

Brown and his colleagues (1962, 1972) are the authors of another impressive piece of social research documenting a key determinant of mental illness. I have in mind their measurement of expressions of emotions ("expressed emotion," or EE) among the families of schizophrenic patients, which, as I mentioned in the previous chapter, is a potent predictor of relapse (cf. Vaughn and Leff 1976; Leff et al. 1983). This line of analysis describes a discrete aspect of social relations that correlates highly with worsening of the course of the most serious of mental disorders. Clinicians are in the process of working out specific techniques to deal with this problem. The special challenge is to develop sharply focused preventive interventions that can be applied systematically to this dimension of the family's response to the sick person in order to reduce chronicity and its consequences. Evidence from intervention studies indicates that this can be achieved (Leff et al. 1982; Falloon et al. 1982).

Other important social influences on health and illness result from a particular birth cohort—the historical experience of persons born at a particular time and the special conditions they face at key developmental stages—which applies demographic constraints on life chances and the life course. Size of an age cohort influences job opportunities, income, marriage, and security in old age. Major institutional and value changes such as deinstitutionalization and alteration of values concerning drug and alcohol use can be shown to exert a direct effect on the types and distribution of mental health problems. An example is the spread of alcohol and drug use among North American adolescents during the past decade with a concomitant increase in adolescent suicide. The current epidemic of violent deaths (homicides, suicides, and accidents) in the United States, much of which is related to alcohol and drug abuse, in 1985 accounted for almost 30 percent of the potential years of life lost under age 65 and an unknown, though perhaps equally impressive, amount of mental turmoil and despair (Centers for Disease Control 1987). Still other important societal forces are social selection pressures, such as one's social class, gender, and ethnicity, which influence who enters psychiatric care, when they enter care, and what care they receive (Mechanic 1986). Psychotherapy is still largely a middle-class phenomenon in North American society; in much of the world it is available only for the elite class or not at all. And the list of social influences is still longer, running from sexual to child-rearing practices, from divorce to child and spouse abuse, from racialism to terror and torture (e.g., in present day South Africa and Latin America), from massive societal transformations that grind people up in the machinery of destruction (e.g., Stalin's Russia in the 1940s and 50s, or Mao's China in the 1960s) to reforms that relieve poverty and protect human rights. Mental health and illness, we may conclude, are inseparable from the social world.

The Stress Model

To account for the influence of the social environment on personality development and the genesis of mental and other disorders, psychiatrists, behavioral scientists, and physiologists developed the model of stress. Although there are numerous formulations and revisions of this model, whose lineaments trace back to the pioneering work of Walter Cannon, Hans Selye, and a generation of psychoanalytically influenced researchers of psychosomatic processes, the central conceptualization has remained stable for decades and indeed has passed over into popular common sense. The homeostasis of the organism is upset by perturbations in its environment. Serious perturbations, or stressors, stress the organism producing a state of strain, which the organism seeks to relieve through coping activities aimed at restoring homeostasis. Those activities, or defenses, may (and often do) either fail to lessen the stress and strain or actually intensify and prolong them, leading eventually to breakdown. Distress and disease, then, result from the interaction of stressors, the individual "host," and the attempts the host makes at adaptation. Stressors are usually modeled as "life event changes" (death of a spouse, loss of a job, divorce, onset of an illness) that are perceived by the individual as "stressful": threatening and uncontrollable to various degrees. These stressful life event changes are said to be "buffered" by the social supports (friends, family, financial and knowledge resources) available to the individual. The outcome of interaction between stressor and supports is a state of the person that is further altered by his coping responses. The contemporary versions of the model go on to assert that life event changes perceived as stressful in the presence of inadequate social support and ineffective coping responses causally contribute to the onset of disorder (medical and mental).

Thousands of studies, ranging from those of caged rats to studies of humans in their natural habitats, provide various degrees of confirmatory support for this model. The findings for a direct causal role in depression are especially convincing (Paykel 1978; Tennant 1983; Ferguson and Horwood 1984; Parkes 1985; Brown, Harris and Bifulco 1985). For other psychiatric disorders the evidence of direct effect is more modest (Rutter 1986), but the association of high stress, low support, and illness onset holds for most psychiatric conditions and for many other diseases as well (Elliott and Eisdorfer 1982; Berkman 1981).

From an anthropological viewpoint, there are a number of troubling aspects of the stress–support–illness onset model. To begin with, stressors and supports are not separable, discrete categories of social variables (Young 1980). Instead, there is a mutually determining relationship between stressors and supports. As components of local social systems, they interrelate systematically. The ethnographer in the family setting or work place finds that yesterday's supports (e.g., a relationship between spouses or daughter-in-law and mother-in-law or supervisor and worker) are today's stressors, and vice versa. Even at the same moment in time a support may be a stressor. Rutter and Madge (1976) demonstrate that stressors and supports become intertwined over time in "cycles of disadvantage" so that they create new stressors and undermine old supports and thereby become a mechanism for cascades of worsening troubles. Stress and support, furthermore, vary inversely with social class so that the lower the class, the greater the stress and the less the support. This is a systemic relationship. That is to say, stressors and supports are aspects of the same local life worlds and the way those worlds are felt and perceived by people. The psychologists and sociologists who divide them into neatly dichotomized predictor variables quantified on different scales are creating artifacts of measurement that lack validity in the patient's life world. Yet this is what is routinely done in epidemiological and psychometric research.

Another problem with this paradigm for studying the influence of the social environment on the sick person is its reduction of a complex, multi-leveled social world into only two dimensions, stress and support. This dichotomy leaves out most of what constitutes social life. Our lives are deeply affected by large-scale macrosocial forces such as the state of the economy, the political situation, social institutional arrangements (e.g., the organizations in which we work, live, and play), and long-duration historical movements that shape our times. There are also cultural conventions and value orientations that assure that certain categories of persons are cynosures (in the North American commercialized culture the beautiful, the athletic, and the rich) while others have stigmatized status. These conventions and orientations lead some categories of persons toward high self-esteem while wounding or damaging the sense of self of others.[3] None of these large-scale macrosocial forces is captured by the stress and support units of measurement.

Nor do those categories describe the dialectical relationship that ties macrosocial processes to personal experience. That dialectic is mediated by the local social system (family, work, community) within which each of us resides. Within a local social system supports and stressors are tightly bound to each other through relationships. In the historical context of relationships with family members, friends, and supervisors and subordinates at work, events are given personal meaning and the social significance they bring to the person is modulated or even transformed. The death of a spouse not only differs from the death of a child as a stressful life event, but the story of the relationship between the deceased and the survivors creates different experiences of bereavement, different modes of meaning for that event. There is a strong tendency in research to configure such meanings of life events as idiosyncratic personal perceptions. While they are that in part, bereavement and other life events are also systematically structured by the history of people's relationships and the local life world within which they are enacted. Think of the death of an 83-year-old retired banker after 45 years of marriage to a 75-year-old woman who survives him. The parents of four sons and daughters and 11 grandchildren, theirs has been a distant, difficult marriage with several separations and years of embittering conflict. The husband has suffered serious chronic illnesses, so that the final decade of their lives together was beset by invalidism, hospitalizations, the menace of having to go to a nursing home, and the slow depletion of savings. The husband dies of complications of cancer that have made him bed-ridden, incontinent, and demented. The spouse's reaction to the loss is relief that at last the suffering is over and even a sense of liberation from the misery of a relationship which she had grown to hate. The sympathy from her children and grandchildren and the sense that in spite of all the burdens of care she stayed the course until the end help shape her experience of bereavement in a different form than that of a 29-year-old secretary, the mother of two small children, whose husband of four years has died unexpectedly in a car accident three weeks after she has lost her job. Now add to these scenarios the macrosocial context: death to a family victimized by the political repression in South America, death of an unemployed black worker during the Great Depression or the civil rights movement of the 1960s in North America, bereavement in an urban slum in northeastern Brazil or the Phillipines, bereavement in the Holocaust. There is a dynamic interaction between historical context, local social system, and personal experience whose structure is obscured and its effects missed when the model of illness onset configures the social world solely as stressor and support. The very terms stressor and support trivialize these social historical realities.

The anthropological model of the relationship of the sick person to the social world is a contextual one that calls for the study of the dynamic interaction we have just described. My research in China attempted to examine both sides of that interaction by studying how the Cultural Revolution, the Anti-Rightist Campaign, and other major political, economic, and cultural changes transmitted powerful sociopolitical effects to individuals which were amplified, altered, or deflected by their local social system (Kleinman 1986). The quality of key interpersonal relationships and one's local status protected some individuals but exposed others to attack and degradation. Exposure of stigmatized persons in one local setting was limited, while in another it was total. The experience of bereavement or job dissatisfaction or illness in one human context was quite distinctive from that in another. The study of this interaction appeared to be a useful complement to the standard assessment of stressor and support.

In another study in which we followed the illness careers of chronic pain patients in Boston over an 18-month period, my colleagues and I learned that ethnographic description of the local life worlds of patients made for more valid understanding of the course of complaints and disability than psychometric measures of stress, supports, and coping. For example, open-ended interviews about loss and the interpretation of its meaning in the lives of our informants frequently disclosed losses missed by closed-ended stress questionnaires, and thereby provided a more accurate assessment of their significance than did a check on a standard self-report form of the degree of perceived severity ranked from $+3$ to -3. Life history and family interviews also revealed that coping is a transaction between individuals in different situations who have relationships with particular histories; it is not a straightforward personality trait as psychological measurements assume, nor is it explicable on the basis of state (situation) alone. The questionnaire quantifies the perception so that statistical analysis can be used to assure a "scientifically" more objective, "harder" measure of significance. Yet the "softer," "subjective" ethnographic description, biography, and local history offer a more valid datum. The scattering of t-tests, chi-squares, and other statistical indices across the pages of a psychiatric article does not a science make. Nor does the interpretation of qualitative findings render a study unscientific. Only in-depth assessments that go beyond superficial responses and gain access to intimate concerns are adequate to the study of how perceived social situations and meaningful relationships relate to illness.

For example, one of the subjects in the pilot phase of the chronic pain study, Mrs. Estelle Wiatt (a pseudonym), was a thirty-nine-year-old administrator in a legal office, the divorced mother of three small children, whose chronic low back pain greatly worsened over a period of six months to the point of keeping her home from work for several weeks. In the course of about ten hours of interviews spaced out during several months, Mrs. Wiatt filled out a standard symptom checklist indicating low levels of depression and anxiety, and answered a stress questionnaire disclosing no stressful life events during the preceding year. In fact, she stated firmly, her emotional reaction was a result, not an antecedent, of the pain, which itself had intensified, she assured me at our first interview, at a time with no greater or different "problems" than there had been since the divorce three years before. "If it is stress-related," she said somewhat defensively, "why didn't my back go out three years ago?"

Mrs. Wiatt described her pain as "terrible." "If it gets any worse, I won't be able to . . . to function at all. I'd rather be dead in that case. Really, I'd think of taking my own life. To tell you the truth, I've thought of it lately." This admission was followed by a burst of tears. I asked Mrs. Wiatt if she felt as depressed as she looked, to which she responded, "It's much worse than I can say. It's so bad, I can't . . . I mean . . . I mean I don't want to talk about it. That's why I didn't check off how terrible I feel on the questionnaire. I didn't want . . . I mean I couldn't face up to it."

"If I didn't have this horrible pain, I wouldn't be depressed," Mrs. Wiatt said. But once she started to talk about the depression, she began to narrate another story as well. For three years, following a deeply upsetting divorce that left her with feelings of betrayal and isolation, this remarkably effective professional woman had been under great pressure as a single parent of three small children who was also deeply committed to her professional work. Her family and closest friends were far away in a small city in the Midwest. With her income and the alimony and child support she received from her former husband, there were no financial problems. But she felt greatly guilty about the two demands on her time: her children and her career, neither of which she felt received the time they deserved.

Mrs. Wiatt believes she coped effectively because her professional work was "a haven" from the drudgery of housework and mothering, from which she felt a strong urge to escape. Her career gave her time away from the demands of child care and the bitter feelings of emptiness and hurt, time during which she was preoccupied with affairs that deeply interested her and that drew her attention away from the worries and unhappiness that beset her. Twelve months before our interview, six months before her back pain became disabling, Mrs. Wiatt's work situation changed dramatically. Two senior partners in the law firm whose affairs she had administered for nearly eleven years retired. Three junior partners were promoted, one of whom was given the responsibility of supervising her work. Her relationship to this partner had never been good. But during the first few months they were forced to work closely together, their relationship deteriorated from "a clash of personalities" to "open warfare." She told me, "I couldn't get along with him. There was no single issue, no explosion. It got worse and worse. Now we are barely able to talk civilly to each other. I can't trust him, and he doesn't like or respect me. Going to work each day is like entering a pressure cooker. I feel like I'm being pressured until I either quit or he asks me to leave. Now I can't stand to be there if I know he will be in the office. He has ruined things for me."

Our talks occurred at a time when there was a downturn in the local economy. Mrs. Wiatt felt she would be unable to find a new position at the same level of seniority, responsibility, and pay. Having devoted 12 years to the firm and to rising to the top of its administrative staff, she did not want to leave under a cloud. Nor could she resign herself to waiting for notice that she had been sacked. To make matters even worse, her former husband had recently been fired from his job as a computer salesman. He had appealed to the court to be released, at least temporarily, from his alimony and child support obligations. "I feel trapped. Now I can't afford to leave my job. But I also can't continue to work under the constant pressure from my boss. Then my pain got worse and worse. The past few weeks I haven't been well enough to go to work."

Whether or not this local social context, reinforced by changing economic conditions, is the major determinant of the amplification of Mrs. Wiatt's pain and the onset of disability, it is quite obviously a very significant problem in her life, a "stressor" if you will. The anonymity of the symptom scale and the stress questionnaire together with Mrs. Wiatt's tendency, at least initially, to deny the seriousness of the nonmedical aspects of her life, led her to minimize her responses on these assessment instruments. Indeed, Mrs. Wiatt told me that she did not mean to disguise her work problem, but the structure of the stress schedule as a listing of discrete events of a stressful kind "didn't make me realize I was supposed to . . . to check off work problem. It isn't my work that's the problem anyhow. It's just one of the partners, who regrettably is my supervisor. I mean you would have to know my story to see the problem."

The approach of the British sociologist George Brown to the evaluation of stressful life events is to insist that the interviewer interpret the subject's story and then fill out the questionnaire for the subject. Of course, this method risks introducing the interviewer's biases; but if properly trained the interviewer will first allow the respondent the opportunity to present and interpret her own story, and only then attempt himself to reinterpret its significance. In Mrs. Wiatt's case, this methodology would have prevented the quantification of invalid information, because it would have allowed the researchers to go beyond Mrs. Wiatt's initial denial to the complexity of her illness narrative. Unfortunately, the vast majority of stress research does not proceed this way. Closed-ended questionnaires and self-report scales provide psychiatric and behavioral science researchers with a quick translation of qualitative understandings into quantitative data. In the process, the meaning of the person's life experience and the nature of the problems in his social field are lost or, worse, mystified. Inasmuch as research with such tools creates the mental health professions' formal knowledge, which in turn is used to train professionals in the professions' orthodox paradigm of practice, it is not surprising that the professions possess an understanding of the contribution of the social environment to illness that tends to seriously underestimate its importance and to obfuscate the systematic workings of cycles of despair.

Cultural Meanings

Most readers may find it easier to appreciate how serious disturbances in social relations contribute to mental illness than to puzzle out the contribution of cultural meanings. I have given one example of this strand in the nexus of influence by describing how disconfirming cultural labels (e.g., the stigmatizing social identity of rightist in China) foster ruinous cycles of generalized hopelessness that undermine one's identity—as in the case of Lin Xiling in Chapter 1. I could also have discussed racialist labels in South Africa, the label of dissident in the Soviet Union, the hidden injuries of the labels of class in England, or the authorization in the past in our own society of marital relations that systematically conditioned women to a label of servitude. Such cultural meanings are a particular aspect of vulnerability to psychosis or dysthymia. As the social psychological literature amply demonstrates, how we view ourselves is a complex evaluation which in part reflects others' expectations and our own anticipation of how others may treat us (Jones 1986). Cultural labels routinize these expectations, so that we have massive confirmation that we, as stigmatized members of a social group, are "disloyal," "unrefined," "inadequate," "appalling"—whatever labels are applied to our particular group. Edgerton (1967) has shown that among the mentally retarded such expectations come to dominate the person's view of himself to such an extent that he feels forced to construct a "cloak of competence" in which he knows neither others nor he himself believes (cf. Langness and Levine, eds., 1986). The sociodynamics of depression, as George Brown and his colleagues

(1978, 1985, 1986) have uncovered them, emerge from such cultural webs of demeaning disconfirmation.

Thurston (1987) offers many deeply moving examples of how stigmatizing labels in China's Cultural Revolution and the negative societal reaction accompanying them induced feelings of guilt, worthlessness, and negative self-identity conducing to despair. Dressler (1985) shows how similarly disconfirming labels may conduce to the onset or exacerbation of hypertension among Southern blacks in the United States. Finkler (1985) does the same for depressed women in rural Mexico. And Waxler (1979, 1981) reasons, as I have noted, that illness labels which are stigmatizing act as a self-fulfilling prophecy to worsen outcome in schizophrenia and other chronic disorders. Goffman [1963] develops perhaps the most complete microanalysis of the interpersonal dynamics of stigma as spoiled identity among the mentally ill, the mentally retarded, and the physically disabled.

But cultural understandings operate in other ways as well. When we are under great social pressure, say, for example, as the result of serious school failure, work conflict, or life crisis such as loss of a spouse, we are shocked out of our ordinary common-sense view of our world and forced to search for alternative ways of making sense of our condition. In traditional societies, religious and moral idioms of distress as well as bodily complaints communicated what was amiss and shaped the social form of distress. Increasingly, in contemporary Western society, the process of modernization has weakened these older forms of dealing with trouble. Although they still are significant channels for expressing problems, they are being superseded by psychological idioms ranging from a general language of stress to more specific existential and affective expressions. These newer idioms convey discontinuities in one's social world not as sin, chest pain, or oppression by the forces of evil, but rather in a language of intrapsychic angst, personal demoralization, and often self-defeating, morbidly introspective hopelessness. There is no scientific evidence to indicate that a discursive, open expression of personal problems as guilt or depression is either more cognitively "advanced" or "healthier" than the other idioms of distress which convey emotion indirectly and through silence, but often with great subtlety and eloquence.

For the anthropologist, the idiom is the symptom. The problem may be misfortune, owing to the obdurate social sources of misery, indistinguishable from similar problems in radically different cultures or historical periods, but the peculiar expression of misery as depression, anxiety, backache, or fear of being possessed results from the particular cultural apparatus of language, perceptual schema, and symbolic categories which constitute distress in one or another mode. Thus cultural idiom orders the interpretation of distress.

Anorexia nervosa, as I have noted (see p. 46), is an uncommon problem in most of the non-Western world, though it is on the increase in Japan.

It would seem to be so tied up with contemporary Western orientations to the female body, more specifically with the role of eating in controlling weight to produce the very slender form that holds greatest sexual attraction and social prestige, that, as I argued in Chapter 3, it can be considered a culture-bound syndrome. That is to say, the cultural meanings of thinness and eating constitute the disorder, albeit psychobiological and family vulnerability factors place certain persons at higher risk for suffering this affliction. Where the body is valued differently and eating conveys meanings other than personal control, obesity will not signify a moral offense or aesthetic blemish; starvation will not be a voluntary choice, but rather an unavoidable fact of life. In such a cultural context, anorexia nervosa does not possess coherence as a local category. Nor does it appear as a behavioral cynosure. Vulnerable individuals may develop a diathesis, but it will be of another form. With the increasing assimilation of Western values among the elite class in non-Western societies, it is reasonable to speculate that, as in the case of Japan, this culture-bound syndrome may increase in prevalence in the most rapidly industrializing of those societies.

Agoraphobia, when not associated with panic disorder, strikes many observers as equally culture-laden. The contemporary Western ambivalence about the proper place for a woman—in the home or in the work force—creates a culturally salient illness experience of houseboundedness that symbolically instantiates a conflict about her own best place (Littlewood and Lipsedge 1987). Agoraphobia does not appear to be a highly prevalent psychiatric disturbance outside North America and Western Europe.

These few examples hardly begin to tap the large store of instances that indicate the contribution of cultural conceptions to the genesis of disorder and the formation of symptom constellations, but they may suffice to illustrate psychocultural process.

There is another side to this subject. Cultural orientations are not limited to laypersons and patients. Practitioners wear theoretical lenses ground from shared cultural conventions as well as from professional values. The practitioner's configuration of the patient's illness problems (e.g., inability to climb stairs to a second-floor bedroom, unwillingness to follow the prescribed treatment regimen, impotence) as problems of disease (e.g., the symptoms of congestive heart failure, the expectable complications of diabetes) is a professional transformation of knowledge. Whether the practitioner takes a more somatic, psychosomatic, or social view of the disease reflects not only the specialty (e.g., internal medicine, psychiatry, public health), but also the clinician's personal distillation of leading models of etiology. Those models reflect strong cultural influence. For example, the stress model is a major model in the popular culture of Western society which has been "scientified" into a professional paradigm. Increasingly in Western societies, practitioners reinterpret bodily distress and its social sources as "psychosomatic" or "psychological" problems (Helman 1985).

Sometimes the latter terms are used to shift responsibility for the patient's failure to get well from the practitioner to the sick person and his family. An exhaustion-weakness-dizziness cluster of complaints, formerly interpreted as neurasthenia, is now diagnosed as depression or a personality problem. This in part reflects the prominence of an intrapsychic viewpoint and the emphasis on individual experience in Western society. The physician's use of a professional label can reconstitute a general health problem, say, prolonged recovery after a heart attack, as a psychiatric one, say, depression. This is much less likely to happen in Chinese society, where the sociocentric value orientation and the very powerful stigma attaching to mental illness discourage practitioners from employing psychiatric labels. Instead, they use medical and moral words.[4]

Chronic pain provides an interesting example of the influence of deeply embedded cultural principles on professional behavior. In North America, chronic pain patients are being rediagnosed as suffering from psychological problems—affective, behavioral, psychodynamic. The practitioner's willingness to identify a behavioral or emotional problem as the source of chronic pain contrasts with his inattention to the political and economic aspects of chronic pain in the redistribution of welfare benefits through an illness test rather than a means test and a disabled rather than a needy role. (Doctors prefer to disregard their role as society's gatekeepers to scarce resources.) Yet these social aspects of chronic pain are well documented and have been shown to be a more powerful determinant of disability than biological or psychological influences (Yelin et al. 1980; Stone 1984; Osterweis et al. eds. 1987). In China and many other non-Western societies, chronic pain has not been separated out as a psychosomatic or behavioral diagnosis, and therefore the healing professions do not differentiate it from other somatic problems. The emphasis on pain as a voluntaristic, individual behavior reflects both the professional orientation of medicine in the West and the influence on medical practice of a value orientation which shifts the burden of responsibility for health from society and the health professions and onto the person, which can result in blaming the victim. This orientation also defines disability heavily in terms of impairment in work performance, in keeping with the main interest of our political economy.

The apocryphal story about the three baseball umpires is an instance of what I have described as the influence of cultural meanings. In this story three retired umpires are reminiscing about baseball. They discuss how they make the decision as to whether a pitch is a ball or a strike. The first, a naive realist, says, "Some are balls and some are strikes, I calls them as they are." "No," says the second, who would seem to have grasped the importance of perception, "some are balls and some are strikes, I calls them as I see them." "No," also says the third, who would seem to have captured the peculiar charm of cultural relativism, "some are balls and some are strikes, but they ain't nothing until I call them!" How an action or behavior is labeled has serious consequences; culture and profession contribute significantly, if more or less tacitly, to the construction of mental illness, a point to which I shall return in the next chapter.

Cultural and Professional Barriers to Prevention

In spite of the evidence pointing to the social origins of depression, the thrust of research is on the identification of its biological correlates, *even if these are secondary*. Biology has cachet with psychiatrists; anthropology and sociology do not. The key item for the biological approach has been "endogenous" psychiatric conditions such as depression, so called because they are believed to arise principally from the psychobiology of the person. This is yet another manifestation of the pathogenetic/pathoplastic dichotomy. As Holden (1986) has pointed out in an article in *Science*, the leading researchers in the field now have impressive data that there is no such thing as depression that occurs solely from biological causes. Endogenicity is refuted by the most recent research studies; and clinicians who treat depressed patients over many years have had the impression that while any given episode of depression in the long course of recurrent depressive disease may not have a clear-cut relationship to environmental factors, the longitudinal course usually offers abundant demonstrations of such a relationship. Yet even the summary article in *Science*, having made the point, fails to follow it up for its preventive and treatment implications; rather it too highlights the very latest biological discoveries.

There is a systematic resistance to dealing with social sources of depression and other psychiatric conditions. Perhaps the idea strikes clinicians as simply too difficult to operationalize in practical programs. Perhaps it also is too threatening, since it suggests that expensive social programs may be more availing in the long run as prevention than the use of drugs and psychotherapy to treat individual episodes of disease (Eisenberg 1987). There is also the unappealing reality that drug companies and psychotherapists derive economic gain and livelihood from the treatment of depression; no particular commercial interests will benefit from preventive programs, in spite of the fact that such programs would contribute importantly to the economy by reducing the costs of one of the commonest sources of disability. There is no effective lobby for social research and sociotherapies to counteract the powerful lobby for biological research and treatments. And the exploitive orientation of the media to the latest scientific breakthroughs assures that biological rather than social issues will receive attention. Even the families of the mentally ill find biological causes more acceptable, since they indicate that mental illness is like all other disorders and they remove some of the burden of guilt. The cultural argument is that this situation is a symptom of the dominant forces in our society and its institutions. In spite of the interests of some psychiatrists and psychologists in social factors and prevention, the orientation of the mental health professions overall contributes to this problem. For psychiatry, the neurosciences hold out the hope of escaping marginality and catching up with the rest of biomedicine (Eisenberg 1986); for psychology, cognitive science and behavioral medicine are the darlings of research funding agencies and hold the promise of financial support for clinical specialists. But the political economy and the cultural system of knowledge production and transformation are the chief determinants of the romance with biology and the devaluing of social science.

Why the social sources of distress and disease have not stimulated a larger discussion among rank-and-file and academic psychiatrists for ways to protect those who are vulnerable to mental illness as well as patients at risk for chronicity is of great interest to students of the psychiatric profession. Social pathology and prevention are often regarded as "inappropriate" for professional researchers and practitioners, since they reach well beyond the narrow focus of professional competence. Here a treatment orientation actively works against a preventive perspective. How the norms of the profession of psychiatry itself contribute to this systematic inattention may take on clearer form in the next chapter when we examine a specific instance.

Perhaps nothing so polarizes the perspectives of anthropology and psychiatry as the question of the effect of large-scale social forces on individual behavior. Many psychiatrists in North America are of a liberal political persuasion that is sensitive to this issue, and this is true of psychiatrists in other societies as well. Yet in the actual practice of psychiatry, especially in bureaucratic institutions that rely on the profession's authorized formal paradigm of knowledge and practice, this interest in larger-scale forces is put aside, as is the liberal political agenda, to be replaced by a focus on the individual patient and at most some concern with his family. The work place, the community, and especially the lines of pressure transmitted via the local social setting from the larger society are outside that professional paradigm. Though it will be argued that mental health professionals have their effect in one-to-one interaction with their patients, where their mandate is for practical interventions, this is not the whole story. Some sociotherapies—e.g., strategies used in comprehensive community care programs to improve employability and teach skills for daily living and reduce isolation and break local vicious cycles—can be applied in clinical settings, but they are infrequently used. Many psychiatrists, moreover, work in the public sector, either in institutions or as consultants to the courts, the schools, and social welfare agencies. In those social settings, they can eschew the model of a one-to-one clinical intervention and work instead with systems analysis and interventions. Few do.

Professional associations of psychiatrists (and also psychologists and social workers) speak for the profession as a whole and lobby actively in the political arena at local, regional, and national levels. They also have access to the media and can marshal public attention. Hence they could be a force advocating specific policies of social intervention. In recent years, the interests of these associations, which for a quarter century following World War II included a consensus for social reform (Grob 1986), have increasingly become economic. Regrettably, the concern of these professional associations has centered almost entirely on the economic situation of their members, which indeed has been eroding, rather than on the economic sources of their patients' problems. Furthermore, as Freidson (1986) notes for professions generally, mental health administrators, teachers, expert witnesses, and members of committees of professional consultants to federal and state government that establish credentials and standards influence the structures of our day-to-day world (if they clearly do not dominate them as Foucault and his epigones aver). Their relative inattention to large-scale social forces, which may begin with the self-serving convention of modern capitalist society to eschew social change as a legitimate activity, doubtless is also enhanced by the specifically North American cultural preoccupation with individual choice, self-help, fear of social assistance engendering passivity, and exaggerated concern with welfare system malingerers. This is less of an issue in Western Europe, where a social welfare system has stronger historical support.

But the barrier in the profession to prevention is also a reflection of the profession of psychiatry's alternative interests; it is not merely a mirroring of societal values. These professional interests influence the creation, transmission, and transformation of the formal knowledge that constitutes psychiatry's professional paradigm for how to understand and respond to mental illness. That is to say, there is a bias in psychiatry in the very way knowledge is created, so that social causes and social remedies are minimized and even denied. Prevention, when thought of at all, is configured as the choices and behaviors of individuals.[5] This bias gains support not only from the way psychiatrists are socialized and earn their living, but from the major sources of support that fund psychiatric research projects.

Anthropology and other social sciences carry the opposite bias. They tend to deemphasize the biological and personal contribution to mental illness, and the value of treatment interventions aimed at curing or caring for the individual. This is simply untenable. The value of creating a substantive colloquy between anthropology and psychiatry is that it draws attention to these biases and can correct them. Social prevention, for example, can only be cost-effective if it identifies individuals under social pressure who are at greatest risk for mental illness because of a combination of psychobiological and social forces. Social revolutions do not do away with mental illness; carefully focused and controlled social change, however, can reduce the burden of risk. The gist of this chapter is that it is useful to integrate social factors with psychobiological ones, not to replace the latter with the former.

In psychiatry, the study of autonomous psychological processes and investigation of person-centered treatment techniques are fundable research strategies. Diagnosis of social pathology and development of societal interventions, especially during the tenure of the reactionary Reagan administration, usually have not been. But there is considerably more to professional interests than this. I turn in the next chapter to consider how the professional paradigm that embeds these interests affects psychiatric practice—in the clinic primarily, but also in the laboratory, the lecture hall, and the administrative suite.

Chapter 5

How Do Professional Values Influence the Work of Psychiatrists?

Psychiatry provides us with the very terms in which our problems are constituted, through its elaboration of the norms and images of healthy mental life, and its characterization of the features of pathology. These enable us to identify what is unhealthy, to classify and measure the problem, and to construe it as remediable. Mental life is now a domain that can be comprehended through, and may be arranged by scientific expertise.

Nikolas Rose,
Psychiatry

Neither domination or impotence may be ascribed to either the professions or their disciplines.

Eliot Freidson,
Professional Powers

Ten years ago, I conducted an ethnography of psychiatric practice in a North American city. Working with several senior clinical practitioners, I observed them practice, interviewed and followed the treatment of selected patients, and collected the practitioners' life histories. I also spoke with their colleagues and with their family members. Since 1980, I have done the same with a much larger group of psychiatrists in China. In this chapter, I draw upon both sets of ethnographic experiences to portray the work of psychiatrists within the ethos of professional values in two radically different societies. The comparison should help differentiate the lines of influence from profession and those from the broader society to the practitioner.

The following transcript is from an audiotape of a North American psychiatrist's initial interview with a patient. The patient, Bill Smith, is a 40-year-old white male physician who works in the hospital where the psychiatrist, Jake Kamin, a 45-year-old white male, also practices. They know each other, though not well, through professional contact. I provide the complete interview followed by a description of the psychiatrist's note in the clinical record. I then contrast these with an entry from the patient's personal diary and a description of how this case will enter the professional literature via an article prepared by Dr. Kamin for publication in a medical journal.

The Clinical Interview*

Bill: I set this appointment up with your secretary as I mentioned on the phone, Jake, to, to . . . to talk about what is going on in my life. Something's wrong, terribly wr . . . wrong.

Jake: Tell me about it, Bill. Start from the beginning.

Bill: The beginning Jake. I mean when was the . . . ah . . . beginning? This thing must go very far back. Way back. But I guess . . . you would say . . .

Jake: Well, why not begin with the way you are feeling now, and when that began, and what it's like? OK?

Bill: OK. I guess its much worse now than its ever been. I . . . ah . . . feel empty, broken, dead to things. I think I . . . I mean I know I'm depressed, very depressed. (Bill Smith starts to cry—slowly and then with increasing force.)

Jake: That's OK Bill, I can see how you feel. It's OK to cry. Tell me about it.

Bill: Oh, gosh, I don't know. It's everything. I just had my fortieth birthday last week, and I . . . I felt so lonely, so dejected. You see . . . I feel disappointed in myself. My personal life, my family, even my career. I've felt this way before, for the last few months, but never so bad. I just felt . . . I, well, I felt there was no sense in going on. (*Bill Smith cries again, though silently now. Jake Kamin puts his hand on Bill's arm.*)

The names Bill Smith and Jake Kamin are pseudonyms to protect the anonymity of the protagonists. For this reason I have also altered identifying details, deleted reference to proper names, and made other small changes in the transcript and in the descriptions of case write-up, diary entry, and research manuscript that follow. In transcribing the audiotape, I did not include all the speech sounds, such as sighs, or mispronunciations, or overlapping speech. To do so would have rendered the transcript too cumbersome to read. I have noted those pauses, "ahs," repetitions, and stutterings which seemed prominent and potentially significant.

Bill: Thanks. I'm OK. What I wanted to say is that . . . ah . . . things got so bad, so bad that I thought I'd be better off dead. I don't mean I would take any action. I wasn't suicidal, only I felt I might just as well be dead.

Jake: I see. It must be pretty bad.

Bill: It is. I feel like things have gone terribly wrong. There's not much left in my marriage. I'm not the father I wanted to be. My research isn't going anywhere. I feel like I made a terrible mistake dropping clinical practice for full-time research. I'm up for a tenure decision and I don't think . . . I mean I know I'm not going to get it. There are other things too.

Jake: And when did it begin to get this bad?

Bill: Oh, about two months ago I started to feel down and very irritable. Next thing I knew I was having trouble sleeping, getting up real early, 4 A.M., and not being able to get back to sleep. Then I started to get very anxious, worried about all kinds of things, frightened. I'm not that kind of person. And our sex life came to an end. She wanted to, but I just had no interest. I gave up the long walks we used to take. I even stopped coming into the lab at nights and on weekends.

Jake: How was your appetite?

Bill: About the same.

Jake: Did you have difficulty concentrating? For instance, on your research, or teaching, or when reading for pleasure?

Bill: I stopped reading for pleasure. And I have had some problem, a kind of slowness reading research papers. . . .

Jake: You mentioned you felt anxious. Can you tell me more about that?

Bill: Well, I began feeling tension. First in my arms and neck, then all over and all the time. I felt like I had drunk too much caffeine.

Jake: Did you have any episodes in which you felt a sense of panic come out of the blue, a feeling of something terrible about to happen, like you might die or lose control or something like that and also felt shaky, sweating with palpitations, tingling, numbness, you know?

Bill: No, nothing like that.

Jake: Which part of the day is worse for you?

Bill: Mornings are. I feel a bit better as the day progresses.

Jake: And you have felt, it seems . . . I mean, helpless, or hopeless?

Bill: Both. I feel hopeless all right. But I don't feel like anyone can help me either. I know I can't help myself.

Jake: Worthless?

Bill: Yeah, real worthless. Useless you could say.

Jake: Have you lost pleasure in things?

Bill: For sure. I don't get pleasure out of the lab work, it's become onerous, a terrible task. Playing with the kids—I used to love to be with them, all I want now is to be alone. Marsha and I don't go out anymore. She wants to; I can't see the point. Even watching sports on the TV; I've lost interest.

Jake: Have you . . . I mean have you had episodes like this before? Before a few months ago.

Bill: Not like this. I'm . . . I've felt down when Dad died last year, but not like this. And I've had some disappointments in the past: grants being turned down, work going poorly, my son John's school problems; but not like this.

Jake: Did you have similar symptoms after your dad died?

Bill: Kind of for the first month or so, then they slowly went.

Jake: Have you ever had any psychiatric problems or treatment?

Bill: Never.

Jake: Anyone in the family?

Bill: Well, Marsha has been seeing a counselor the last few years. Maybe that's part of the problem. She has changed so much. She's more independent. Seems to love me less. And spends less time with us. I've been taking more care of the kids and the house.

Jake: How about your folks, or sibs or the wider family?

Bill: Sorry, I don't get you?

Jake: I'm asking if there is a family history of mental illness or depression?

Bill: No, no one. I mean John, my son John has had dyslexia . . . I guess that's some kind of psychiatric problem. But not serious problems.

Jake: Go ahead, I interrupted, I'm sorry, you were telling me how you feel.

Bill: Yeah! I'm not so sure there's much more to say. I feel . . . I feel depressed and irritable, angry, and I've been having headaches. I've had sinus headaches for years, but they've gotten bad again in recent weeks.

Jake: Any other symptoms with them?

Bill: No. And they aren't all that bad, or different than before.

Jake: And it all started?

Bill: That's the thing, Jake. I'm not sure when it all began. I'd say two or three months like this, but only this bad the last month or so. Before that . . . well, let's see. My father died a year ago last month. The anniversary was pretty tough. That upset me a great deal at first. All those archaic feelings returned. You know what I mean. You remember back to when you were a kid. All those feelings of love, disappointment, hate. I mean we had a . . . complex, ambivalent relationship . . . And it all came back last month and things got much worse. But there are other problems that made me feel bad even earlier.

Jake: All of that is important and we want to get into it later, but are you saying you began to feel depressed after your father's death and it just got worse and worse? Before I thought you said the symptoms disappeared for a while, then came back?

Bill: Not exactly like that. I grieved and then it wasn't so bad, but it kept coming back. The sleep and energy and depression disappeared until a few months ago. Troubled and ambivalent feelings . . . ah . . . about my dad went away, came back, went away; but other things were going on also.

Jake: Like what?

Bill: Things have been bad with Marsha for years. We have been married fifteen years. Everything went pretty well the first five years. Then when we first moved here, ten years ago almost, I got so very busy with my work we grew distant to each other. She had the three kids and the house and the dogs, and her parents were getting old and sick, and then John developed the learning problem. Marsha always had wanted to go back to school, but there . . . there wasn't any time. And then . . . well, then . . . then I had an affair. Nothing very serious. But I had a college student as a lab tech and we were there in the lab at night and on weekends. We . . . well we started becoming lovers. Then Marsha found out. All hell broke loose. She, I mean Marsha, threatened to kill me and herself and the kids. I mean she went after me with a kitchen knife, screaming that I had ruined her life. She was in her nightgown and her hair was all wild and she was wild, crazy. She threatened to leave. She did leave for a few days. I came back to my senses. What was I doing playing around with a college student and ruining my family?

That is when . . . ah . . . the rot set in. Things have never been the same since. I guess its my fault . . . yeah, it was my fault. I hurt her . . . bad, and our marriage too.

Jake: And that has continued up to now?

Bill: I'm not sure what you mean by continued. Things got better for a while. Then we started having fights. Marsha got depressed, blamed me, went to see a counselor, then another, the one she is seeing now. She began to change. She went back to school, spent less time with me and the kids. We became distant. Not much of a sex life. It always had been good up till then, but over . . . over the years it's kind of died. Now we don't have any. Ironically now she is more interested than me.

The last few years we have had other . . . ah . . . concerns. John's school problem has gotten worse. And he's real aggressive with the other kids. Marsha and I have fought a lot over time and responsibilities. She rightly wants more time, time to study [*she is in a doctoral program in art history*] and to be by herself. Well, that means I have to stay with the kids and I should be in the lab or traveling to meetings. It has had a real effect on my work.

When my father died, well it all came to a head. She took it very hard too. I left for a few days. Or she kicked me out of the house. We had a big fight one night after being at a party. I drank a bit too much and I guess got angry at her. She threw all those things up to me. How I had ruined our marriage. Ruined her chances. Hurt the kids. Even John's problem. Then she told me I never loved anyone, not . . . not even my father. I . . . I lost my head. I slapped her and pushed her around. I cried and cried and asked her to forgive me. But she went wild again. She told me to leave. So I packed up—I think it surprised me even more than her—and left. I went to live in a small rental apartment for a few weeks. It was terrible, desolate, empty. I spent all my time blaming myself, feeling guilty and ashamed. And I kept thinking how she said . . . ah . . . I never loved my dad. Then I begged her to let me come back. To start over. But the rot was there. Do you know what I mean? It never was the same. She was cold, distant. She said I had hurt her too much. Me . . . I also felt distant. Something had spoiled our marriage.

Jake: I'm sorry to break in Bill, but you mentioned that the fight started after you had been drinking. Has alcohol been a problem?

Bill: No, no. I have a drink now and again. But not often. After my dad's death I got drunk a few times—once at that party, an . . . another time when I was by myself in the rental apartment.

Jake: Go ahead.

Bill: Well, there's not much more to add.

Jake: You said earlier that you are upset about your work, your research.

Bill: Yeah. You know I'm forty. When my birthday came around, I looked back on all the things we talked about. And I began to see that I hadn't achieved what I wanted, what I expected to. It's hard to talk about this. I know you're a psychiatrist . . . but you're also an academic, and a very productive clinician and administrator. Full-time research is different. You only do one thing. Well, me . . . I started out like a house on fire and then slowly over time, it petered out. I haven't made any major discoveries. My best work is five or six years behind me. Oh, I get grants all right to keep the lab going, and I have a few trainees of real quality. But the ideas, the original ideas—they don't come like they used to. And I haven't done what I wanted to. I always wanted to make a major discovery, a major breakthrough. Nobel Prize quality. That was my fantasy. I drove myself to do it. I felt I had to. All my life was taken up in my work, and daydreams about a signal success. Something so important everyone would honor me. I guess a lot of us come to see that it isn't going to be that way. That the dreams we have are not to be realized. That we have come to middle age only to discover we are not . . . ah . . . what we thought we were. Then there is disappointment and loss—yes, a real sense of lost opportunities, lost direction, even the future is obscure. And we ourselves, what? Much less brilliant, less powerful . . . less energy and less everything than we thought we had. How then to live . . . to work? As a second-rate academic? Just holding on until the race is run? I'd never been that way. But all of a sudden I felt like my courage had slipped away. I felt terribly lonely. My Dad, he . . . he was a failed inventor. He was supposed to be brilliant. But nothing much came of his inventions. He got bitter and old. And I had the feeling he thought my mother and I regarded him as a failure. I saw the same thing for me. I never worried about tenure before. All of a sudden I could see that I might not get it. Why give it to someone who clearly is not nearly as productive as he once was? The field I feel is . . . ah . . . moving beyond me. I'm . . .

Jake (interrupting):   This is all very interesting and important Bill, but I need to ask you some things specifically before we finish up today. OK?

Bill: Okay, I was just trying to give you an idea of what has been happening. . . .

Jake: You mentioned earlier feeling it would be better to be dead. Have you made plans to take your life or been preoccupied with suicide?

Bill: No. I'm not suicidal.

Jake: But you did say you'd rather be dead? Or rather you felt that way?

Bill: Sometimes. But not now. And I've never thought of seriously taking my life or made plans.

Jake: Could you tell me if you did make such plans?

Bill: I think I could, but I haven't.

Jake: OK, OK. Let me ask you about thoughts you may have had recently. Have you had any strange thoughts, like belief your body was rotting or that you had a serious medical problem?

Bill: No.

Jake: I'm trying to get at any delusions.

Bill: No, none. In some ways I think depression has made me see things more clearly, more honestly with less self-protection.

Jake: No hallucinations or suspicions?

Bill: No; none.

Jake: During this period or before, ever had any manic symptoms? You know, grandiose thoughts, hyperenergetic, giving away money, thinking you were very special?

Bill: No, no mania. I wish I had more energy. I always thought I was special, don't we all? But as I said, my problem seems to be not that idea but . . . but beginning to feel the opposite that I'm not as special as I thought.

Jake: Anyone in the family with depression?

Bill: No, I already said no one, except for Judy.

Jake: Bill, you said your father's death really affected you greatly?

Bill: It did.

Jake: Was he depressed before he died or in the latter part of his life? I ask because you said he was bitter.

Bill: Well, he seemed lonely, easily hurt, and disappointed. I don't think he was depressed like I am now. But he wasn't happy or optimistic.

Jake: Did he have any particular symptoms before he died?

Bill: He died from a CVA and he had had a few episodes of syncope and frequent headaches.

Jake: I see. You mentioned your ambivalent feelings about him. We can talk about these next time in detail, but can you briefly tell me what you meant when you used the word "ambivalent"?

Bill: Well, just that. I loved him. He was my father. And I have lots of warm feelings about him. But I also have negative feelings. He was a real Puritan. A taskmaster. Driven and driving. He had such ridiculously high expectations of me. And he seemed never satisfied. And then he seemed . . . at the end I mean . . . such a failure. I had the feeling that was me too. That somehow he had set us both on a disastrous course.

Jake: And these were the ideas that kept coming back?

Bill: Yes.

Jake: And they are still strong now?

Bill: They are.

Jake: Do you feel that this depression could be a thing that grew out of your grief and the difficult feelings you had for your . . . your dad?

Bill: I guess . . . guess so. I hadn't thought of it only that way. I . . .

Jake: The anniversary of his death seems to have really affected you.

Bill: It did. The whole thing came back along with all the other things going on in my life. But I felt just like when he died.

Jake: Well, I think that does it. You can see as well as I that you've got a major depression. Now depression is a treatable disorder, a biological problem. We have excellent meds for it, and I think we should start one now. I want to talk to you too about the things you mentioned, especially your father's death, because that could very well be connected. I mean short term . . . that is, a few sessions of psychotherapy can really help, but meds are what will get you getter. Now, have you had any allergies or bad reactions to drugs?

Bill: No, but I know you need to take medication for this condition. I'm willing to do it, but I want to talk to someone about all these things I feel . . . pent up inside. I've never talked to anyone. I feel the need to talk it out. I know you guys think its a brain disorder, but whatever it is, it's so deeply affected my life, I need to deal with these things. Is that the kind of thing you do, Jake?

The interview continued for another five minutes, while Drs. Kamin and Smith agreed on a course of a tricyclic antidepressant drug and weekly psychotherapy sessions for five or six weeks. Below I record Dr. Jake Kamin's note in the clinical record as he wrote it down immediately after Dr. Bill Smith left the office.

The Write-Up in the Psychiatry Record:
The Professional Construction of a Case

40-year-old white male physician with several months of depression, hopelessness, helplessness, anhedonia, irritability, guilt, insomnia, and energy and concentration disturbances. Associated anxiety. Not acutely suicidal but has had some suicidal thoughts. No plans. No delusions or hallucinations. No family history. No prior episodes. No mania. Sinus headaches, chronic, amplified by depression. No other medical problems. No alcohol or drug abuse.

Bereavement 13 months ago following death of father. Grieving with ambivalence and modeling of father's symptoms seems to have extended into depression. Depression deepening over past few months, with greatest increase over past month since anniversary of father's death. Worse past month. Work, marital, family problems contributory.

Impression

Axis I: Major Depressive Disorder secondary to bereavement (prolonged and pathological).
Axis II: No personality disorder.
Axis III: Chronic sinus headaches.
Axis IV: Severe bereavement reaction, 4/5.
Axis V: Reasonably good level of functioning, some work-related problems and chronic mental tensions, worsening. But able to cope.

Plan*

(1) Doxepin, begin at 50mg, bring up to 150mg qhs over course of 1 week
(2) A few psychotherapy sessions to do grief work.
(3) ENT consult to rule out serious sinusitis and? CNS effects.
(4) See in 1 week.

                                        Jake Kamin, M.D.

---

*Doxepin is an antidepresssant; qhs means each night at bedtime. ENT stands for an ear, nose and throat physician. CNS is central nervous system (i.e. the brain).

Patient's Diary

That night Dr. Bill Smith returned home and wrote a lengthy entry in his diary, from which I have selected the brief excerpt printed below.

> I don't think he heard me. I wanted him to listen to me not for the diagnosis but for the story, my story. I know I'm depressed. But I wanted him to hear what is wrong. Depression may be the disease, but it is not the problem. The problem is my life. "The center doesn't hold. Things fall apart." It's falling apart. My marriage. My relationship with my kids. My confidence in my research. My sense of purpose. My dreams. Is this the depression? Maybe it caused the depression. Maybe the depression makes it worse; or seem worse. But these problems also have their own legitimate reality. This is my life, no matter if I am depressed or not. And that is what I want to talk about, to complain about, to make sense of, to get help to put back together again. I want this depression treated, all right. There is something more I want, however. I want to tell this story, my story. I want someone trained to hear me. I thought that was what psychiatrists do. Someone ought to do it, ought to help me tell what has happened. But all he seemed interested in was the diagnosis and my dad's death. I'm sure that is part of it, but so much else is going on. I need to talk to someone about my whole world not just one part of it.

Professional Discourse

Dr. Smith's "case" entered the official professional discourse on two occasions. Dr. Smith became part of the aggregate statistics that Dr. Kamin reported to his psychiatric colleagues at a case conference as cases in his practice of major depression secondary to bereavement. In that presentation Dr. Smith's name did not appear. But in several of the slides, he was described as one of the cases reported by Dr. Kamin. In these slides, Dr. Smith's insomnia, lack of energy, guilt, and anhedonia are catalogued along with other vegetative complaints of depression. He is left out of the cases with suicidal plans or suicidal acts. But he is included in the cases with significant anxiety symptoms and those with anniversary reactions during which they experienced symptoms that the deceased had experienced. Although details of his bereavement response figure in the aggregate figures, little else from his life history is measured or counted.

Dr. Smith's case also appears in the aggregate statistics Dr. Kamin cites in a manuscript that he has prepared and plans to submit for publication to a professional journal. In that professional paper, Dr. Smith's case is used along with many others to support Dr. Kamin's conclusions about the relationship of bereavement to depression. Dr. Smith's story is written up as a brief vignette illustrative of Dr. Kamin's thesis that bereavement is an important cause of depression, and that anniversary reactions play a special role in the progression of bereavement into clinical depression. A paraphrase of the vignette goes as follows:

> Dr. X is a 40-year-old white male with symptoms of major depressive disorder. Symptoms of grieving recurred in the tenth month of bereavement and greatly worsened at time of the anniversary. One month later a full-blown DSM-III major affective disorder was present, and he made his first contact with a health professional. Although many of the same symptoms were present the first month after his father's death, they diminished over the next six months before exacerbating. At the time of the anniversary reaction, Dr. X described characteristically "archaic feelings," including disturbing images from childhood and feelings of love, disappointment, hate, and the complexity and ambivalence of their relationship. Dr. X experienced bad headaches, which his father had experienced prior to the CVA that caused his death. He attributed the exacerbation of his depressed symptoms to the anniversary reaction as well as other problems in his life. Dr. X also complained of the same feelings of loneliness, emptiness, dejection, and self-disappointment that I have described in the preceding cases, and which his father, like the fathers in the other cases, also had experienced in his final period. Like those cases too he had a great need to see all aspects of his life as affected and affecting him. And indeed there were other significant recent life event stressors in his marriage, family relations, and work (including multiple losses, real and symbolic) along with inadequate social support and self-defeating coping.

The Role of Professional Norms in Clinical Work

Dr. Kamin is a senior clinician, board-qualified in psychiatry, something of an expert in the treatment of depressive disorders, especially clinical depressions complicating bereavement, for which he has a well-deserved local reputation. He is a forty-five-year-old white male, who at the time he treated Dr. Smith was in the midst of difficult divorce proceedings with his wife of sixteen years over the custody of their three children. Dr. Kamin is on the clinical faculty of the department of psychiatry at the medical school, which means that he is out of the tenure track for full-time researchers and in a special track for part-time medical academics who are principally clinicians and clinical teachers. He administered, at the time of the interview, a subunit in a division of the department of psychiatry in one of the medical school's affiliated teaching hospitals, the hospital where Dr. Smith's laboratory is located.

Dr. Kamin's own father died five years before, during a period when he was experiencing marital problems. Although he never sought treatment, in retrospect he believes he became depressed for a period of months following the anniversary of his father's death. Like his father, who died of a heart attack, Dr. Kamin experienced chest pains at the anniversary, pains that were severe enough to make him feel he too was suffering a heart attack. The medical evaluation convinced him he was not experiencing a heart disorder, but rather psychosomatic symptoms symbolically related to his father's death. From that time he began to specialize in this problem. Dr. Kamin has been greatly influenced by the literature on this theme. He believes that helping patients grieve their real and symbolic losses is what psychotherapy for complicated bereavement is about. Dr. Kamin also has strong convictions about what constitutes competent professional practice in the diagnosis and treatment of depression.

"Before giving a dynamic or behavioral or social interpretation of depression, it is essential to do as good a job at description of the symptoms as possible so that you get the diagnosis right. I'm first and foremost a descriptive psychiatrist, and I see my first task as getting the phenomenology right. If that leads to a diagnosis of a treatable psychiatric disorder, say, major depression or panic disorder or manic-depressive disorder or schizophrenia, then the next step is the prescription of specific medication. For after all this is a disease of brain and endocrine system."

"I prescribed Doxepin for Dr. Smith, and after six weeks he was symptomatically very much improved. We spent four or five sessions talking about his life problems and especially about his father. I got him to grieve. Then when things looked much better, I referred him for longer-term psychotherapy. You know, to deal with other problems in his marriage and work. But frankly, at that stage my thinking was he no longer was suffering from depressive disease. I don't feel Dr. Smith was completely satisfied with our visits, even though he thanked me for the symptomatic improvement. I think he had a lot to get out and work through. I sent him to someone whom I felt would do a good job on that aspect of things, the life problems and kind of midlife crisis. (I don't like the term, but that's what it amounted to.) Frankly, I haven't heard further from him or his therapist. I've been so busy I haven't had time to really think about him until today."

Later in the same interview, Dr. Kamin told me that after the grief-oriented short-term psychotherapy, he felt Dr. Smith had no further need for psychotherapy. He made the referral for long-term therapy only because Dr. Smith insisted that he do so.

The structure of the initial interview illustrates a point made earlier in this book: Dr. Smith presents *illness*—a chaotic mixture of symptom complaints, coping responses, life problems, his own interpretations—and out of this patient-centered narrative Dr. Kamin configures a psychiatric disease. He does this by organizing the interview to provide answers to questions that are based upon the diagnostic criteria for making a psychiat-

ric diagnosis of major depressive disorder. He also rules out, through these
questions, other clinical hypotheses: psychosis, alcoholism, manic-depressive disorder, and an organic mental disorder related to sinusitis. Along the
way he listens intently for certain kinds of data, most notably those which
confirm his theoretical speculation concerning the relationship of depression to bereavement. The patient feels that in constructing the disease, Dr.
Kamin has neither fully elucidated the anguish of his illness experience
nor allowed him to express the range and depth of the problems that beset
him. Dr. Smith does not feel that the turmoil in his life story is being heard.

From a professional perspective, Dr. Kamin's evaluation is likely to be
viewed positively by descriptive psychiatrists but not nearly so positively
by those with greater interest in the process of psychotherapy. The former
are likely to see his clinical work as competent, the latter as at best marginal. Indeed, I suspect most psychotherapists would criticize Dr. Kamin
for just those interrogative interventions that obstruct the flow of the patient's account which descriptive psychiatrists would regard as essential in
applying rigorous diagnostic criteria to define a disease. (Psychotherapists
would also criticize Dr. Kamin's lack of self-reflexive insight into the personal source of his own interpretive "interests," i.e., countertransference.)

It is important that Dr. Kamin rule out suicidal intent. After all, clinical
depression for a small but significant percent of patients is a mortal disorder. If not properly assessed, tragedy may result. It is also important that
he interrupt the patient's life narrative to determine if a treatable disorder
is present. An "unconstrained interview," without interrogation or inter-
ruption, might do justice to the patient's life story but would be a serious
and dangerous impediment to the evaluation and treatment of the disease.
Somehow, the psychiatrist has to do both. Conflict among therapists centers on what constitutes the proper balance.

In his case description, academic presentation, and written report, Dr.
Smith's case undergoes even greater reduction. It is fit into a framework
to support Dr. Kamin's main thesis; but left out are all those areas of his
patient's life that to the patient and doubtless to readers with a different
conceptual framework would seem essential. The reduction to an aggra-
gate statistic seems to do an injustice to the subtle complexity of this life
story. It would seem to lack validity not because what Dr. Kamin writes
isn't true, but because the context of Dr. Smith's life is left out and the
vignette seems a distortion organized around a single determinative cause.
After all, a family therapist might see the marital difficulties as the chief
and earliest source of Dr. Smith's later problems. And a developmentally
oriented psychiatrist might emphasize the career conflict and midlife stress
(cf. Lazare 1973; Gaines 1979). Finally, there is the fiction that all scientific and professional presentations commit in which findings are presented
in "objective" terms that leave out contradiction, alternative possibilities, and self-reflective aspects of the case (Mulkay 1981). For example,

Dr. Kamin's personal experience of past grief and of pending divorce would seem to significantly influence those answers he regards as significant and those he appears to disregard. He constructs the evidence to fit his concerns; whereas I could reconstruct the case in a rather different way as an example of a tightly integrated vicious cycle creating demoralization and amplifying distress.

The movement from illness to disease to case report and onward to research knowledge is a movement of social construction guided by professional norms of how to conduct an interview, what to regard as evidence, how to sift and marshal that information to support a clinical judgment, and how to write up a typical case and research article. This construction is indeed constrained by the patient's experience. Dr. Kamin neither fabricates that experience nor is insensitive to it. Within that constraint, however, there is ample opportunity to develop the "case" in one direction or another. Personal experience of the practicing psychiatrist both in the clinic and in his home influence that direction, as Dr. Kamin's life situation illustrates. Professional norms, moreover, are not a simple reflection of a homogeneous professional system shared by all members (see Freidson 1986). Dr. Kamin is primarily a practitioner. His job is to apply the official knowledge of his profession to individual cases. That always involves a transformation of what Freidson calls "formal knowledge" into "working knowledge."

Dr. Smith, in contrast, is a researcher, a creator of new knowledge. That knowledge also undergoes change in moving from the laboratory to the research literature (Latour and Woolgar 1979) and from that literature into textbooks. In the course of this transformation, the uncertainties, controversies, and fragmentary nature of research data are ironed out and a "classical" textbook picture of a case of a given disease emerges with a consistency, simplicity, and total structure quite at odds with both the messy research findings and the "blooming, buzzing" confusion of real life as lived by a particular person. For the practitioners who further rework this knowledge in the crucible of practice, it is essential to recognize both the transformed nature of the textbook presentation and the metaphoric leap between that formal knowledge and the working knowledge fashioned in experience.

Dr. Kamin is also a clinical administrator, and as such has a responsibility to his institution (the teaching hospital where both he and his patient practice) that cross-cuts his professional interests. The administrative and research side to professional norms become especially powerful in organizing a treatment plan. Here clinical experience, model of psychopathology, and professional psychiatric values concerning the possibility and significance of suicide are intensified by Dr. Kamin's administrative responsibilities (he feels compelled to do something quickly for a member of the hospital's professional staff for whose psychiatric problems he feels a special medical responsibility) and by his research interests (he is collecting cases to investigate depression following bereavement) to urge rapid and technically powerful "biomedical" treatment with an antidepressant drug and the use of psychotherapy in a highly delimited, short-term mode. Dr. Kamin told me later that in treating medical colleagues, it is important to impress them with the biomedical side of psychiatry, about which he feels most are suspicious. Thus, treatment becomes an opportunity for raising the specialty's marginal status in the profession and that of his clinical unit in the hospital. This plan conflicts with Dr. Smith's wish for existential confession and life course review—and it is not the only effective way to treat depression.

Individual practitioners are influenced to treat patients in a particular way not only by their institutions and their personal interest but also by the school of psychiatry to which they feel allegiance and by the official standards set by their professional association. Psychiatry is split into often irreconcilably opposed "schools"—biological, psychoanalytic, behavioral, social, and so forth. Each school has its own institutional centers, its own academic luminaries and rank-and-file members, and its own journals, meetings, societies, and "classics." Each school teaches a different view of human nature (cf. Schwartz 1986) and a distinctive value paradigm for professional practice (cf. Gaines 1979, 1982). The "classics" are journal articles and books that set out the latest information in distinctive formats, in keeping with each school's ideology, for researchers, students, and the lay public. What holds these schools together is the professional organization of psychiatry into a national association (the American Psychiatric Association) that lobbies for its members' interests in national and local political economies and that influences such key questions as licensing and, together with the American Board of Psychiatry and Neurology, another national association, the setting of standards of practice. The last few years have made explicit what has long been a less openly admitted function of the national association—namely, to protect the control of its members over a specially sheltered sector of the market, the treatment of mental illness (cf. Freidson 1986). But the shelter is not complete, and the association's influence is not determinative. Other professions—psychology, social work, and a myriad of forms of psychotherapists—contend for their market share. The association's influence is indirect, through the agencies of federal and state governments, the courts, via numerous consulting committees, and more recently through a wide variety of publications and public relations efforts which aim at influencing public opinion.

The profession's influence is greater than this sketch suggests, however. Through its official diagnostic criteria (DSM-III), the profession provides the formal standard for assessing psychiatric disorder that is used by the courts, by the disability system, and in clinical work generally. It is upon this official taxonomy of formal knowledge that Dr. Kamin draws to interpret Dr. Smith's disease and to justify its treatment. The American Psychiatric Association is now planning a manual of treatment that will specify the range of appropriate treatments for mental illnesses. That manual could codify treatment much as DSM-III codified diagnosis. Because of sharp disagreements among psychiatrists over which therapies are most suitable, which provoked fears that the psychiatrist's legal right to prescribe would be restricted, it should come as no surprise that this treatment manual has stimulated intense debate over whether its status should be official or not. At the APA's Annual Meeting in 1987, it was decided, in deference to the strong opposition, that the manual would be unofficial (Jonathan Pincus, personal communication, May 11, 1987).

It is all too easy to point to the potentially dark side of treatment standards and regulations without acknowledging their positive contribution. After all, in the absence of standards, practitioners are licensed to treat according to their own therapeutic biases and remunerative preferences. We are all too familiar with the results, i.e., unwarranted surgery, endless psychotherapy, therapeutic fads, and so forth. There is a genuine dilemma between useful and flexible standards that protect the public and rigid regimentation on the basis of received wisdom that locks both care giver and patient into an iron cage of orthodoxy. This dilemma is sharper now for all professions, not just psychiatry. And the problem almost certainly will become worse in the 1990s, because of a broad societal movement toward ever more elaborately refined standards.

It is important, as Freidson (1986) cautions, not to overemphasize the power of the profession. The patient, his social circle, public opinion, and other professional (primary care, psychology, social work) institutions and bureaucratic (the hospital, the HMO, the university) organizations influence psychiatric practice, as our case illustrates. The profession, moreover, incorporates spectacular diversity. Other psychiatrists would have responded to Dr. Smith rather differently. And the patient leaves the encounter still very much the master of his fate. At its worst, professionalization of Dr. Smith's life problems produces insensitive and inhumane treatment. At its best, it assures technically competent help with remediable problems. Much of the time it falls somewhere in between.

The profession is also not the only influence, as we have seen, on the practitioner. Personal experience and institutional concerns are often very influential. Shared cultural orientation also plays a role. It is inconceivable that Dr. Smith would have expressed his personal problems as fully if he were a member of a non-Western society. Rather, his headaches might have provided him with a more indirect somatic idiom for expression and response to his social problems. (This occurs frequently even in our own society.) The patient's responses offer resistance to the practitioner's orientation, resistance that often turns the treatment of different patients in unpredictable directions. For example, Dr. Smith, though a laboratory researcher, will not accept a solely biomedical explanation (and treatment) for a problem he believes emerges from his life situation. Nor is he as convinced as Dr. Kamin is that the chief causative factor is grief following his father's death. He insists on referral for long-term therapy—a form of care Dr. Kamin feels is, in this kind of case, unnecessary and in general ineffective. Because of his patient's urging, Dr. Kamin makes a referral he would not otherwise have made.

In this complex mélange of interests, however, professional norms do exert important effects, ones often hidden to the practitioner. While too anxious a concern with reflection on the nature of that influence may conceivably paralyze the psychiatrist as a clinical actor, too much denial blinds him to pressures which are not always in the best interest of patient care. Dr. Kamin is deeply interested in Dr. Smith's disease; he is not as concerned with Dr. Smith's illness experience. For the patient, particularly if he suffers from a chronic condition, the opposite is often true. Overly narrow and routinized professional medical standards of how to technically treat depression, the disease, may dehumanize the patient (and the practitioner). Care organized by such standards can be ineffective or even contribute to the downward spiral of demoralization. A medical perspective may restrict the sphere of intervention to too limited a target. Treating the problem as a social tension in Dr. Smith's relationships, or in fact, as a cultural one, in Dr. Smith's American upper-middle-class professional world, might encourage a broader set of interventions applicable to the treatment of a class of similar cases: such as marital counseling, family therapy, counseling on academic issues, legal referral, or psychotherapy that explores adult developmental conflicts. These interventions may even offer opportunities to prevent the long-term consequences of the cultural pressures that beset many mid-career professionals like Dr. Smith. The historical development of the psychiatric profession has witnessed transformations in the salience of the patient's narrative and the diagnosis of the disease for the clinical construction of a therapeutic approach. (Scull, ed., 1981). At present the pendulum is swinging away from the former and more toward the latter.

In the seventh chapter I will return to explore this tension between medical and social perspectives in psychiatry by examining what relationship psychiatry should have to social science. Before ending this chapter, however, I wish to offer a comparative example of the influence of professional and societal values on clinical practice by drawing from the studies my wife and I have conducted of the vicissitudes of the psychiatric profession in China.

Psychiatry in China: The Practitioner, the Profession, and the State

The year is 1983. My wife and I are observing patient-doctor transactions in a psychiatry clinic of a teaching hospital located in a city in south central China. The room we are in is a cement rectangle, 15 feet by 10 feet. There is a long table at one end, with two young psychiatrists sitting on opposite sides. Each is interviewing a patient. Behind the patients, both of whom are women in their thirties, are their husbands as well as two other patients (and their family members) who are waiting their turn to see the psychiatrists. The two interviews proceed simultaneously. I am listening to Dr. Li (pseudonym), a 33-year-old postdoctoral fellow who is specializing in the clinical care of patients with neuroses, interview Mrs. Wu (also a pseudonym), a 35-year-old mother of a six-year-old who stands fidgeting by her side. Mrs. Wu is tall for women in this part of China. Her height, together with her harsh, clipped accent, indicates that she is from the north. She is an accountant in a nearby factory. Her husband—a balding, obese cadre in the same work unit who is eight years older than his wife—stands behind their daughter, anxiously shifting his weight from one leg to the other. I am doing all I can to concentrate on this conversation, because the one proceeding 5 feet away together with the general level of noise in the clinic are a constant distraction.

Dr. Li has just concluded five minutes of interviewing Mrs. Wu about her symptoms. She has complained of fatigue, lack of energy, dizziness, difficulty falling asleep, and a troubled, anxious feeling—all of several years duration. He has taken her blood pressure and felt her pulse. He has also read through her clinic record, noting that, though this is her first visit to the psychiatry clinic, she has been seen frequently over the past three years in the hospital's internal medicine and Chinese medicine clinics, where she has received a wide variety of drugs and other somatic therapies (*qi gong*, a traditional breathing and relaxation technique, acupuncture, massage, etc.) for neurasthenia. Dr. Li has already asked Mrs. Wu questions about the symptoms of depression, anxiety, and phobia; he has learned that she has symptoms of generalized anxiety disorder.

Dr. Li: Why are you so nervous?

Mrs. Wu: I've been this way for the past four or five years. Before that I was a calm person.

Dr. Li: How did it begin?

Mr. Wu: Suddenly, for no reason.

Dr. Li: For no reason?

Mrs. Wu: Well, our family has not been peaceful. My husband's mother lives with us. She is old and irritable. We argue almost every day. Since she left my brother-in-law's apartment and moved in with us, five years ago, not a single day has gone by when she doesn't complain about me, my daughter, the cleaning, the cooking, the way I treat my husband . . .

Mr. Wu (breaking in):   She is old! Old people are demanding. We must be more tolerant. After all, she is my mother.

Mrs. Wu: I have tried to be tolerant for five years. Look what it has done to me. I feel troubled and unhappy all the time. We argue and then I feel even worse. I argue with you and with Meiwen *[their daughter]*. It makes my neurasthenia worse. Some days I feel too upset to go to work.

Dr. Li: Do you and your husband disagree over this problem?

Mrs. Wu: Yes! He sides with his mother. He will not consider sending her back to live with our brother-in-law. He wouldn't take her back anyhow. My sister-in-law wouldn't agree. Her husband listens to her . . .

Mr. Wu (breaking in again):   We cannot send her away. Where would she live? Who would take care of her? I am the oldest son, this is my responsibility. Even the leaders of our unit agree.

Mrs. Wu: Yes, Old Yang and Wei tell us to endure. They have not been of any help.

Dr. Li: Yet, what they say is true. She is your family member. It is your responsibility to care for an old mother-in-law. Perhaps it is your neurasthenia that makes you irritable and stubborn. It interferes with your duties as a wife and daughter-in-law.

Mrs. Wu: That is the problem! The neurasthenia makes me feel troubled and agitated. I can't bear her complaints. Because I am sick, I am irritable and argue with my husband too and even my daughter. Can you give me something for the dizziness and fatigue?

Mr. Wu: She is right. Because of this disease, she is not the same. She cannot tolerate stress. She must rest. But my mother is always complaining that she is not strong enough, not doing enough. Surely it is the neurasthenia.

Dr. Li: No problem. We will give you some Valium and a Chinese tonic for this disorder. Then you will feel better, and the family problem will become easily resolved . . .

Mrs. Wu (interrupting):   Valium is no use! I have taken it many times. Don't you have a stronger medicine for my nerves?

Dr. Li: All right. We can use a new neurological medicine. A more powerful tranquilizer. That should make you calmer and relaxed. We also have a biofeedback machine that may be of use. If you can return next week, we can try it and also see how the medicine worked. In the meantime, strive not to argue with your mother and husband and daughter. You must contain your anger. You know the old adage: "Be deaf and dumb! Swallow the seeds of the bitter melon! Don't speak out!" Once the disease is better, your relationship with your mother-in-law will improve. But in the meantime you must work hard at not making things worse. Understand?

Mrs. Wu: I understand. But what about my tiredness and lack of energy? I am too weak to work. I need rest.

Mr. Wu: Yes. Even the leaders say she should rest at home.

Dr. Li: I will give you a note for your work unit, recommending that you be allowed to rest at home for a week. But only one week.

Mrs. Wu: Thank you! Then I may really feel better.

The interview ended after Dr. Li wrote out the prescriptions and the note to the patient's work unit. He also asked Mrs. Wu to return in one week for a trial of biofeedback. In the patient's chart, he wrote a very brief, four-line summary of the physical symptoms, the diagnoses (generalized anxiety disorder and a chronic personality problem), and the prescribed medications. Having completed this transaction in 12 minutes, he turned to the next patient.

If we compare Dr. Li's interview with Mrs. Wu and Dr. Kamin's interview with Dr. Smith, both of which are initial assessments by psychiatrists of outpatients with neuroses, we see several of the key differences that distinguish the practice of psychiatry in China from psychiatry in North America. In China, the practice of psychiatry, for all but perhaps the elite class, is public, family-centered, and more medical than psychotherapeutic. Dr. Li takes Mrs. Wu's pulse in part because this act has great significance in Chinese society, where it is the icon of classical medical practice. Rather than explore the psychodynamics of Mrs. Wu's symptoms and family problems, Dr. Li accepts the patient's presentation of daughter-in-law–mother-in-law conflict as the salient psychosocial problem. After all, this paradigmatic conflict is traditionally recognized as a core tension within families in Chinese culture, and it is also discussed in the standard Chinese psychiatric texts as a prototypical precipitating factor in neurasthenia and other neuroses.

Perhaps most surprising to a North American therapist, Dr. Li gives voice, within ten minutes of meeting the patient and her husband for the first time, to a strongly moralistic exhortation in support of traditional, sociocentric, Chinese values concerning the filial responsibility of adults for the care of elderly parents. He does so after seeing that this is a source of conflict between Mrs. Wu and her husband, and after learning that the leaders of their work unit have already given voice to this traditional moral injunction. Dr. Li's clinical method is not psychotherapeutic in the accepted Western sense, nor does he recommend psychotherapy as a treatment alternative. The central therapy is medication, in addition to which Dr. Li provides a medical excuse for the patient to take a week off from work—a prescription which both the patient and her husband have actively sought. But Dr. Li does practice a medical form of psychotherapy. He offers the patient and her husband a sanctioned medical explanation for their conflict—namely, the effect of Mrs. Wu's neurasthenia on her personality and relationships—which they are quick to accept. That explanation does not hold Mrs. Wu, her mother-in-law, or her husband at fault. Rather it reinterprets their family conflict somatopsychically as the result of a medical disorder.

Dr. Li, who is one of only 3,000 or so physicians with some level of training in psychiatry in China, has not arrived at this style of practice intuitively. He has observed physicians of all kinds, including senior psychiatrists, perform this way, and he has read about it in textbooks. He is aware that Mrs. Wu and her husband will find his approach acceptable, indeed that they expect him to proceed as he does. Nor would Dr. Li understand the criticism of Western psychotherapists that he has neither explored the full context of potential psychosocial problems (e.g., work, marital, or sexual issues) nor obtained a "deep" understanding of Mrs. Wu's personal experience. Twelve minutes for an initial psychiatric assessment will strike North American psychiatrists as rushed and inadequate. Yet it is close to the average for patient-doctor interactions by Dr. Li's colleagues.

Probably, many readers will find Dr. Li's evaluation of Mrs. Wu "superficial." When I have presented cases like this to fellow psychiatrists in the United States, that has been the usual response: "How superficial!" Psychiatry in the West is strongly influenced by implicit Western cultural values about the nature of the self and its pathologies which emphasize a deep, hidden, private self. In contrast, both classical Chinese texts and the contemporary common-sense viewpoint among Chinese, both laymen and psychiatrists, affirm that the self is chiefly interpersonal. The Chinese view the self, to a large degree, as consensual—a sociocentrically oriented personality that is much more attentive to the demands of a particular situation and key relationships than to what is deeply private. That is not to say Chinese have no private side to their individuality. They clearly do. But for Chinese psychiatrists and patients that intimate domain is not as important as is the immediate field of social ties and practical moral problems (Hsu 1971; Bond, ed., 1986). Social context, not personal depth, is the indigenous measure of validity. In such a context, moral exhortations, not psychologic interpretations, are viewed as the core rhetorical task of persuasion and healing.

For this reason, by the way, the model of the self in psychoanalytic theory, or any other professional therapeutic psychology, seems to me a serious distortion when applied to Chinese (or Tamils, Javanese, Japanese, Hausa, or others) who are not acculturated to Western values or socialized into Western paradigms of personhood. In order to do justice to the salient psychodynamic processes among Chinese (or Tamils, Javanese, Japanese, Hausa, or others), we require a different psychoanalytic theory. Such a theory should include seemingly universal psychological processes—perhaps repression and transference but also key concepts from other professional systems of psychology for which there is evidence of cross-cultural validity. To this should be added a very large measure of what is unique to the structure of the self (and its pathologies) in Chinese culture—for example, an inner censor for group consensus, a drive to harmonize complementary oppositions, e.g., ambition and loyalty, a developmental emphasis on filial obligations, intensive training in an ego ideal of moral self-cultivation, great sensibility to the tactics of shame in interpersonal negotiation, subtle idioms of self-expression based on bodily metaphors and the use of silence, perhaps a distinctive version of psychosexual development with less intensity to its conflicts and even unique complexes, among many other differences (for a hint of what this might mean in Japanese culture see Doi 1986). The interpretation of psychodynamics also would be different, then, and so would the rhetorical techniques through which such psychodynamic formulations are therapeutically applied in psychotherapy.

Dr. Li's experience of the self, his intuitive grasp of the dynamics of other selves, and his clinical work, I insist, arise from an interplay of these universal and culturally particular elements in psychology. Our evaluation of his practice—and of our own—must take this particular mixture into account if our assessments are to have cross-cultural validity. Because they fail to do precisely this, much of psychoanalytic psychology (and other Western-based psychologies as well) is inapplicable in its present form to Chinese. And indeed, this is how the vast majority of Chinese psychiatrists and psychologists regard it. In fashioning their own professional psychology, it is to be hopped, Dr. Li and his fellow mental health professionals in China will help identify those aspects of our professional models that are culture-bound to the West along with those elements in indigenous Chinese models that may have cross-cultural validity.

The origin of psychiatry in China is not Chinese medicine, which, though it recognized madness, hysteria, depression, and psychosomatic effects, neither set out a separate branch of knowledge on mental illness distinct from the rest of medicine nor trained a group of specialists to treat the mentally ill. Nor is the origin to be found in late-nineteenth- and early-twentieth-century medical missionaries like Dr. John Kerr, who built the first modern psychiatric hospital in Canton in the 1890s. Rather the development of psychiatry only began in the 1930s, when R. S. Lyman, an American psychiatrist trained by Adolph Meyer, built a major training center in neuropsychiatry at Peking Union Medical College, where he developed a broadly eclectic tradition, and Fanny Halpern, a Viennese neuropsychiatrist, taught the subject at several key institutions in Shanghai (see Kleinman 1986). Between them, these two expatriates trained the first generation of indigenous psychiatrists, a number of whom would develop academic departments in Chengdu, Changsha, and Nanjing as well as in Shanghai and Beijing. The students of this first generation of Chinese psychiatrists head the profession and its institutions.

After the chaos of the Anti-Japanese War (1937–45) and civil war (1945–48), the stability and optimism ushered in by the early years of the Communist state witnessed the flourishing of psychiatry along with the medical profession generally and the other professions. The anti-American sentiment of the Korean War years and the Stalinism of the 1950s, however, substituted Russian neuropsychiatry, particularly Pavlovian psychology, for North American and Western European orientations. During the Anti-Rightist Campaign in 1958, psychoanalysis came under specific attack as an unacceptable example of Western bourgeois influence. Nonetheless, the 1950s, in retrospect, are viewed as a near golden age in the development of the profession, a period of rapid growth of psychiatric research and mental hospitals. All of this came to a complete stop in the early period of the Cultural Revolution (1966–76). Intellectuals and professionals generally were assaulted and degraded. The fledgling professions of psychiatry and psychology were particularly hard-hit targets. Mental illness was attributed, by the ultraleftists, to wrong political thinking. Psychiatric hospitals were seized by revolutionary committees—psychiatrists cleaned toilets, toiled in communes in distant rural areas, worked as ordinary primary care doctors, or were imprisoned. A number, under great pressure of public degradation ceremonies, committed suicide. While there is no evidence of systematic abuse of psychiatry in China to imprison dissidents, as occurs in the Soviet Union, during the chaotic years of the Cultural Revolution patients went untreated or, worse, underwent political reeducation for delusions and hallucinations.

The past ten years of societal rebuilding and rapid economic development have been a time in which all the professions have revived and reprofessionalized.* Psychiatry has modernized rapidly. The old Russian neuropsychiatry has been jettisoned. New American, European, and Japanese influences are felt through returned scholars and students, the visits of for-

---

This section draws on materials previously published in Kleinman (1988).

eign experts, and the reopening to the international professional literature represented by a flood of foreign books and journals which for three decades were banned. Chinese psychiatrists are engaged in the international intellectual ferment of a discipline whose biological, psychological, and social paradigms are generating extensive empirical research and reconceptualization of psychiatry's basic ideas. This ferment is more varied in China owing to attempts to integrate traditional Chinese medical concepts.

At the present time, there is remarkable decentralization. No official system of diagnoses is recognized. Each of the major centers is in the process of developing its own system, as is the national organization. But in the latter, in contrast to the past, there are now heated debates over new formulations. This is an impressive change in a centralized society where psychiatric listings determine disability, competence, and other social statuses.

Institutionally, the major change in the professions is the assertion of professional control over the academic and clinical work units. Psychiatrists are replacing political cadres as the administrators of psychiatric hospitals and research centers. But the secretary of the local branch of the Communist Party still is the most powerful force in these institutions, making key decisions such as those concerning promotion. Loyalty to the work unit challenges national and international professional ties, and also discourages collaboration across units. While China does not yet have "schools" of psychiatry, the major centers for training and research have defined particular spheres of interest—epidemiology, biological psychiatry, social rehabilitation, etc. One small unit has even developed a program in psychoanalysis.

The practitioner's experience in the Chinese system is greatly different from that of his North American counterpart. Few medical students freely choose psychiatry. Rather they are selected by their schools' leaders and told they will become psychiatrists. A practitioner enters a hospital after medical school and may stay there the rest of his professional life, moving up from trainee to junior physician, senior psychiatrist, chief of a service, and director. Because the work unit is a total institution where he and his family reside, eat their meals, raise their children, and develop their closest friendships, the practitioner is extremely sensitive to the concerns of the unit's leaders and staff. Because of the history of criticism and attacks on intellectuals, the professional members of a work unit are careful to note which way the wind blows and bend with it. Practice is shaped, then, as much by local norms as by national professional and cultural preoccupations. There is a tension between institutional and professional loyalties. Within professional institutions there is an additional tension between returned scholars and students with a strong Western orientation and those more resistant to Western models. The persistence of the Chinese medicine tradition and the continuation of 100 years of attempts to marry imported technology to Chinese values encourage the idea of developing a truly Chinese psychiatry—a phrase widely expressed but rarely defined.

Dr. Li's experience of clinical work has been shaped by this milieu. He is a graduate of the medical school where he currently practices, a former trainee in its psychiatry training program, and now a postdoctoral fellow and junior staff physician. Although he is up to date on DSM-III and ICD-9 and also on the latest psychopharmacological drugs, he finds certain Western models of psychosocial care inappropriate and therefore does not keep up with this subject. A behavioral rather than a psychodynamic treatment method strikes him as clinically appropriate. He is also sensitive to the fact that the senior psychiatrists in the clinic are invested in biofeedback and have bought an expensive machine, one they wish to see used. And Dr. Li knows that both the patient's unit's leaders and the hospital's cadres will support a medical request for one-week sick leave with full pay, but not one for a longer period. These various levels of clinically relevant knowledge include Dr. Li's intuitive understanding of what his patient and her husband expect of him. That sensibility is informed by cultural as well as professional sensitivities which lead patient and doctor to replicate a paternalistic Confucian model, but one in which patient-oriented negotiations take place indirectly or under the subterfuge of professional hegemony.

Freud somewhere said that when the patient enters the analyst's office, at least four people are in the room, since the patient's transference to the practitioner based on parental models conjures the ghost-like presence of his mother and father. For Dr. Li and his colleagues, the room is filled with live people. But present as well are the ghost-like apparitions of the leaders of his and his patient's work units. Those images of cadres bring the Communist Party and therefore the state into the clinic. Because their discussion is public, without confidentiality or legal protection of either the physician's or the patient's rights, both Dr. Li and Mrs. Wu are extremely cautious about what they say and do. In fact, Dr. Li told me he did not approve of granting patients like Mrs. Wu a medical excuse for sick leave. He felt it was unnecessary and might even encourage chronicity and provide secondary gain for disability. Yet he did not want Mrs. Wu, her husband, or their unit's leaders to complain to the hospital's administrative cadres, a common practice which in the end, he knew, would get the sick leave through the "back door" and cause trouble for himself and his colleagues.

Dr. Li, who has spent half a year at a leading psychiatric center in North America, also is critical of his department's official support for the concept of neurasthenia. Although he has conducted research to show that this diagnosis is not as therapeutically useful as the new DSM-III taxonomy, he joins in the consensus because his senior colleagues support it, his patients expect it, and the secretary of the local branch of the Communist

Party warned him after his return not to act as if only Western concepts and methods were useful. While participating in the consensus, he uses any occasion he finds appropriate to lobby for his point of view. He became particularly vocal during the few months of intense demands for democratization in late 1986 which preceded the student demonstrations and the campaign against "bourgeois liberalization" that they provoked. Subsequently, he has again become more circumspect about his individual point of view.

Each week, on Tuesday afternoons, there is a political discussion in Dr. Li's department, and each month the hospital's medical staff holds such a meeting. During the Cultural Revolution these meetings, which occurred more frequently, were tense confrontations, during which criticism was leveled at the professional staff by workers, cadres, and fellow (usually lower-level) professionals. In recent years, the meetings have become pro forma discussions of national policies like "the four modernizations," in which professionals like Dr. Li no longer feel the pressure to demonstrate revolutionary zeal. Nonetheless, at times these meetings are the occasion for the secretary of the local branch of the Communist Party and his staff to question the direction the professional directors of the hospital's subunits are following, and thereby to reassert publicly the primacy of the political system. For Dr. Li, who usually jokes about them, these meetings are a still menacing reminder that his profession is not autonomous, that the political apparatus of a totalitarian state diffuses into the everyday work of the professional. Nonetheless, political control is moderated by an increasingly assertive profession, which has produced a creative tension in the modernization of China's psychiatry and its other professions.

China's profession of psychiatry is struggling to achieve a space that it can control within the tight constraints of the Chinese political system. During its worst period, as we have seen, the profession was nearly destroyed, to the detriment of patient care. Yet even in the dark time of the Cultural Revolution neither the political apparatus nor the professional institutions forced physicians like Dr. Li to participate in the most extreme abuse of psychiatry's ethical standards. That has happened elsewhere and is an ever-present threat in many societies, where psychiatry has become a major modern institution of social control. The influences of professional and cultural values, which I have examined in daily practice in "normal" settings, extend along a continuum to more extreme situations. I think we must at least briefly consider the systematic abuse of psychiatry by societal and professional powers—an issue of great significance in our time. For it is precisely in our epoch that psychiatry has come to play a key role in torture, terror, and political repression generally. Thus, after analyzing the effect of values in the routine care of patients, I think we must confront those extreme situations in which the profession becomes the tool of societal forces in the genesis of inhumane treatment and unquestionable evil.

Coda: The Societal and Professional Abuse of Psychiatry

"Walter Schellenberg, the head of the German Foreign Intelligence Service, paraphrased a report Heyde [Werner Heyde, a Nazi psychiatrist] wrote on Georg Elser, the carpenter-electrician who nearly succeeded in assassinating Hitler in 1939, describing it as the 'best analysis' made at the time, and revealing to us how far psychiatric corruption could go:

'[Heyde] said that the assassin was a typical warped fanatic who went his own way alone. He [Elser] had psychotic compulsions, related especially to technical matters, which sprang from an urge to achieve something really noteworthy. This was due to an abnormal need for recognition and acknowledgment which was reinforced by thirst for vengeance for the alleged injustice which had been done to his brother [who had been arrested as a Communist sympathizer and sent to a concentration camp]. In killing the leader of the Third Reich he would satisfy all these compulsions because he would become famous himself, and he would have felt morally justified by freeing Germany from a great evil. Such urges, combined with the desire to suffer and sacrifice oneself, were typical of religious and sectarian fanaticism. Upon checking back, similar psychotic disorders were found to have occurred in Elser's family.'" (Lifton, 1986, p. 118)

Heyde and the other Nazi psychiatrists held an evangelical belief in the Nazi racialist ideology, especially in the mystical notion of a biological state free of racial impurities like Jews. The Nazi doctors committed heinous crimes against humanity that are all too easily explained as the actions of depraved individuals. But it is important to remember that rank-and-file German psychiatrists as well as luminary academic psychiatrists at Germany's prestigious universities, who have exerted a powerful influence on the profession's formal knowledge worldwide, consented to the Nazi program and participated in the atrocities with very little protest. As Robert Lifton shows in his amazing study *The Nazi Doctors*, they responded to the idealism, especially the biological romanticism, and the terror the Nazis used to quiet dissenters, and carried out daily actions that went directly against basic medical ethics, not by brutally irrational, idiosyncratic behavior, but by conscientiously following what they regarded as the paradigm of appropriate professional and scientific work. In Heyde's clinical account of Elser, we see the use of psychiatric categories and clinical reasoning to turn Elser's act of political resistance into pathology. This is a shocking instance of medicalization. What Lifton has discovered is that the entire Nazi apparatus of murder in the death camps was organized under the legitimation of biomedicine and with the active participation of doctors (see also Hanauske-Abel 1986). That is to say, terror, torture, and mass homicide were medicalized.

In 1933, shortly after Hitler and his Nazi Party came to power in Germany, the psychiatric profession capitulated, first to Nazi orders that schizophrenic, mentally retarded, and epileptic patients be sterilized, then to the medical murder of the institutionalized mentally ill. Hundreds of thousands were killed—by lethal injections, deliberate sedative overdoses, prescribed starvation, and eventually by gassing. Psychiatrists played a daily role in the selection, prescription, and actual delivery of these "therapies." Psychiatric hospitals became the first killing stations, before the death camps. Lifton convincingly demonstrates that the medical killing of the disabled psychiatric patients became the prototype for the Holocaust.

The Nazi ideology of Aryan superiority, of the degeneracy of other races (like Jews), and of the need for racial purity and the consequent belief in a murderous eugenics authorized by "life unworthy of life" became part of the everyday clinical judgment and therapeutic practices of the German psychiatrists. This routinization of evil is surely psychiatry's darkest hour. But it is not entirely unparalleled. Psychiatrists and other doctors in certain South American societies are regularly involved in torture. The profession of psychiatry in the Soviet Union and other Eastern European societies has become the major system for political oppression of dissidents (Bloch and Reddaway 1977). Even in China, during the Cultural Revolution, psychiatrists were largely silent when their patients were relabeled as exemplars of wrong political thinking and were taken out of the protection of the hospital and exposed to psychological and physical abuse.

Nor are the abuses of psychiatry limited to totalitarian societies, though by far the worst excesses occur in such settings. At a lesser level of abuse, the professional values of psychiatrists in America who work for the CIA or the military are subordinated to priorities that are frequently at odds with those of professional ethics. Indeed, triage in battlefield conditions in military medicine runs directly counter to peacetime professional medical standards, because a conscious decision is made to leave the sickest for last. In those settings, the professional's values are transformed to serve bureaucratic and institutional interests. I don't contest the legitimacy of such transformations of values in times of war or other national emergency; yet I do believe the routinization of institutional and other nontherapeutic priorities can run counter to the interests of patients and humane care. I believe this can (and, more often than we accept, does) happen in large institutions of all kinds—VA hospitals, for-profit hospitals, HMOs, and so forth. I am familiar with the potential and real abuses that emerge when Japanese psychiatrists, as another example, keep patients in for-profit mental hospitals after their illness has improved, without due process or informed consent, because family members prefer institutionalization, money is to be made, and the government is willing to collude in this abuse of involuntary confinement (Munikata 1986; Stone 1987). For these reasons, I am in disagreement with the American Psychiatric Association's protest to the UN Center for Human Rights' report *Principles, Guidelines and Guarantees for the Protection of Persons Detained on Grounds of Men-*

tally Ill-Health or Suffering from Mental Disorder (Psychiatric News, January 16, 1987), which has the self-serving ring to it that the profession knows best how to regulate its members and protect its clients, even though I find that report extreme and biased. The profession must not be the sole arbiter of its ethical and technical standards, any more than the state should. Psychiatric care can benefit from an appropriate degree of internal and external oversight. The question is to find the right mix and the practicable method.

Clearly, there is an enormous difference between the Nazi crimes and the abuses that occur in contemporary North America and Japan. From the anthropological perspective, however, both are at different ends of the same continuum of abuse. The working psychiatrist makes clinical decisions or engages in therapeutic practices that are shaped by societal and professional values. Those values can be made to serve inhumane interests and can also create inhumane practices.

The implication for the profession and for the practicing psychiatrist is that the structure of professional ethics may be overtly corrupted or tacitly undermined. The Nuremberg Code of Medical Ethics—and other international systems of medical ethics—provide some protection against the more heinous abuses. But as the reports of Amnesty International abundantly document, such protection is limited. For the anthropologist this is a classic instance of the social fact that psychiatrists, like all professionals, are members of political systems whose ideologies and institutional structures shape the conditions of work and the knowledge applied to such work.

There are several kinds of structures that can and do limit the abuse of psychiatry. Perhaps two are most significant. Various mechanisms for the expression and resolution of lay grievances assure that even if the profession as a whole comes to condone inhumane treatment, patients and families can still, should public opinion be unable to change things, have recourse to alternative agencies, e.g., the courts, to have their cases assessed. International professional standards and their local review, including review by professionals from other regions of the country and from international organizations, can be helpful, Nonetheless, we are all aware that these structures are fragile, easily subverted, and only partially successful. Ultimately, the question of abuse of psychiatry is one of the relationship of a particular practitioner in a particular situation to a particular social system. This is an eternal question as pertinent to Socrates as it is to us today. It is a question of morality as personal experience. The modern exemplar, for me, of the psychiatrist's moral choice to be authentic to his role as a healer, even when he is under the greatest pressure toward abuse of that role that a modern state can muster, is Anatoly Koryagin (1987). A Soviet psychiatrist, nominated for the Nobel Peace Price, who was held for six years, until recently, in the most appalling circumstances in the prisons of the Soviet Gulag for his defense of the mental health of dissidents and his criticism of the abuse of Soviet psychiatry, Koryagin has held fast to his "doctor's conscience . . . by my calling, I was obliged to restore health and not to ruin it" (Satter 1987; p. 3).

The perspective of social science cannot wish this moral problem away either as a social, not individual, issue or as one that can be addressed only at the political level, though the political level is absolutely crucial to this question; that perspective can be drawn on to increase personal sensibility to this problem by encouraging in the practitioner a self-reflective stance toward professional and societal values as they influence his clinical decisions and actions. I take this to be an example of the utility of anthropologizing the practitioner's gaze. That anthropological sensibility should encourage a routine scanning of one's professional perspective in light of alternative perspectives—the patient's, the family's, other professionals', other cultures'. This approach cannot assure courageous moral action; it can, however, establish in the practitioner's daily behavior a mechanism for routine moral reflection.

Chapter 6

How Do Psychiatrists Heal?

There are many ways and means of practising psychotherapy. All that lead to recovery are good.

Sigmund Freud,
On Psychotherapy

What makes the majority of Indian approaches to mental health different from the dominant Western view on the subject, however, is their emphasis on the relational. In the Indian prescriptive lists . . . one is struck by the number of ideals of mental health that prescribe the person's behavior in relation to others, especially family and community. A restoration of the lost harmony between the person and his group . . . was one of the primary aims of the healing endeavors in the local and folk traditions.

Sudhir Kakar,
Shamans, Mystics and Doctors

The method of the art of healing is much the same as that of rhetoric.

. . . then this is the goal of all his [the rhetorician's] effort; he tries to produce conviction in the soul.

Socrates,
in Plato, *Phaedrus*

During recent years much has been made of the somatic therapies employed by psychiatrists to treat mental disorders. Compared with the psychopharmacologic agents available before the 1950s, there has indeed been great progress. Drugs are now available that can control flagrantly disorganized psychotic behavior, relieve the immense distress of uncontrollable

108

panic, and greatly reduce the suicidal desperation of profound melancholia. Lithium can limit the profoundly disruptive swings to mania and depression in patients experiencing that bipolar diathesis. But there are some reasons for disquiet as well.

By and large, the types of pharmacotherapeutic agents used today have been around for several decades. Refinements have been made, but in spite of the advances in knowledge of neurophysiology and neurochemistry, no new "breakthroughs" in practical psychopharmacology have advanced the therapeutic efficacy of the clinician. Even more unsettling is our current awareness of the dire side effects of long-term treatment with the most potent of the psychopharmacologic agents. The proportions of the tragedy of tardive dyskinesia—a movement disorder of disfiguring lip smacking and grimacing caused by long-term use of antipsychotic drugs—are only now becoming fully apparent, and the extent of their medical-legal and ethical consequences is still not clear. The withdrawal hypothesis, mentioned earlier in my discussion of Warner's (1985) work, is a provocative thesis that the chronic use of drug therapy contributes to the chronicity of schizophrenia; it will keep researchers active for years to come and, if found even partially correct, will radically change the clinical consensus on the treatment of the most severe of the major mental disorders.[1]

Compared with antibiotics and other disease-specific therapeutic agents used to treat acute medical diseases, antipsychotic and antianxiety drugs are clearly not "magic bullets" that eliminate disease causes. The antidepressant drugs come the closest to this therapeutic fantasy, but they are ineffective in at least 20 percent of cases, are associated with significant relapse rates, take weeks to achieve their effect, and are equaled in efficacy by at least two types of psychotherapy (Boffey 1986; Holden 1986). Psychiatric drugs are more like palliatives and anodynes used to reduce symptoms in chronic medical disorders (e.g., asthma, psoriasis, arthritis) for which there are no complete cures. Most serious mental conditions require long-term drug use to treat repeated recrudescence of symptoms. Patients may be impressed by the list of psychopharmacologic medications, but primary care physicians or specialists in internal medicine, who are accustomed to an enormous array of therapeutic agents, are often surprised by the relatively limited drug therapies with proven efficacy available for the treatment of psychiatric conditions. I do not mean to say that drugs are unimportant in psychiatry—far from it. I only wish to correct the widely popularized but, to my mind, grossly exaggerated impression one can get from the media that drugs have so revolutionized the practice of psychiatry that adequate psychiatric care is essentially the handing out of pills.

For the internist and the surgeon, what distinguishes psychiatric treatment from the rest of medicine, besides the relative weakness and limited range of its somatic therapies, is its use of "talk therapy." Primary care practitioners such as family doctors and nurse practitioners, to be sure, not infrequently practice a kind of rough and ready supportive psychotherapy without explicitly calling attention to it as such—some without fully recognizing that they do so. Not all psychiatrists, of course, practice psychotherapy, and indeed most psychotherapists are not psychiatrists. Nonetheless, in the West, psychotherapy of one kind or another is practiced by most psychiatrists, and most patients go to psychiatrists with the expectation that they will participate in some kind of talk therapy. Perhaps of even greater significance, psychotherapy is closely associated in the minds of the general public with what psychiatry is all about. In North America, where there are more psychiatrists than in all the rest of the world, psychotherapy also occupies a central place in the profession of psychiatry's self-image of how psychiatrists should provide care for their patients. Indeed, it is not at all uncommon in North America to observe an academic psychiatrist conduct laboratory research for a large part of the day, then put aside his laboratory coat and step into his office to see several hours of therapy patients. The anthropologist is struck with the cross-cultural differences in the salience of psychotherapy. In Europe and especially non-Western societies, psychotherapy is much less central a component of psychiatric care.

Economic reward contributes to the salience of psychotherapy in psychiatric care. For Blue Cross and other third-party health insurance agencies that pay for that care in the United States, much of what they reimburse psychiatrists' outpatient billings for comes under the broad and fuzzy definition of medical psychotherapy, whereas other physicians usually do not receive reimbursement for this form of therapy. Finally, in the profession's textbooks and academic colloquia on treatment, the question of how the psychiatrist heals is most often configured as the problem of how psychotherapy heals. That is because even biologically oriented psychiatrists are sensitive to their professional audience's tendency to equate the words "therapy" and "healing" with psychotherapy.

Long dominated by psychoanalysis, psychotherapy is today a huge but fragmented field of practice. Besides the better-known psychoanalytic, behavioral, cognitive, existential, interpersonal, and counseling "schools," there are hundreds of the most different kinds of practices that go by the name psychotherapy (Herink 1980). The term "psychotherapist" stands for an equally bewildering array of persons, running from members of the allied professions of psychology and social work to pastoral counselors and a very wide assortment of laypersons—those who practice art therapy, dance therapy, music therapy, co-therapy, telephone therapy, charismatic and many other forms of religious healing, polarity therapy, dozens of kinds of meditation and relaxation therapies, EST, other group treatments, hypnosis, and much more besides. Indeed, in the United States there are about 35,000 psychiatrists, more than 60,000 fully trained psychologists, and under 100,000 licensed social workers, but there may be as many as 1 million unregulated lay therapists!

For purposes of defending their market share, psychiatrists bill third-party payers under the code: medical psychotherapy, which in theory unites the specific medical skills of the psychiatrist with knowledge and skills in conducting psychotherapy. But there is no agreed-upon standard for defining what in practice a medical psychotherapist is supposed to do (Goleman 1986). Excluding the prescription of drugs, which in the event some psychiatrists refrain from prescribing when "doing therapy," it would be extraordinarily difficult to distinguish what a physician-psychotherapist does from the treatment provided by his nonphysician colleagues. There is no evidence, furthermore, that the type of professional degree influences the outcome of psychotherapy for patients (Smith, Glass, and Miller 1980). The remarkable findings in most studies of psychotherapy outcome are, first, that psychotherapy appears to be effective in the treatment of a wide range of conditions, and, second, that its efficacy does not seem to be greater for any particular school (Luborsky, Singer, and Luborsky 1975; Strupp, Hadley, and Gomes-Schwartz 1977; Smith, Glass, and Miller 1980; American Psychiatric Association Commission on Psychotherapies 1982; Williams and Spitzer 1984). Nor does level of professional training or even extent of experience seem to significantly influence outcome (Rioch 1966; Uhlenhuth and Duncan 1968; Durlak 1979). There are also conditions that are not responsive to psychotherapy, e.g., organic brain disorders, and there are toxicities of psychotherapy, though they are less numerous and serious than those caused by drug therapy (Bergin 1975; Hadley and Strupp 1976).

A recent multicenter clinical trial, funded by the National Institute of Mental Health to study the treatment of clinical depression, showed that cognitive psychotherapy and a mixed psychodynamic-interpersonal modality were equally as effective as antidepressant drugs (Holden 1986). Even though these talk therapies take longer to work and therefore are more costly, the findings have been interpreted by psychiatrists and other psychotherapists as a vindication of the use of psychotherapy. The development of methods to apply psychotherapy to marital relationships, family ties, groups of patients, outpatients in primary care clinics, and a new array of medicalized social problems from rape to bereavement and other forms of "post-traumatic stress disorders," premenstrual syndromes, menopause, midlife crises, and even unemployment has further intensified interest in the revitalized talk therapies. Furthermore, although more research is needed, psychotherapy appears to be cost-effective in reducing the utilization of general medical services, prescription of psychoactive medication by primary care doctors, and hospitalizations (Mumford et al. 1984; Borus et al. 1979; McGrath and Lowson 1986).

One of the more interesting controversies in the psychotherapy field is the question of whether the effects of psychotherapy are due to specific or nonspecific agents of change (Strupp and Hadley 1979; Karasu 1986). Each school of psychotherapy claims that unique elements in its technique of practice are responsible for specific therapeutic effects (see, for example, Wolpe 1958; Beck, Rush, et al. 1979; Klerman et al. 1984). Outcome research conducted by adherents to a particular school tends to support these claims (e.g., Rush et al. 1977). But overall the empirical evidence fails to demonstrate specific effects of specific techniques. Rather it points to nonspecific, shared aspects of psychotherapy as the most likely chief determinants of efficacy (Frank 1974; Karasu 1986; Torrey 1986). Later in this chapter, I will return to this research for assistance in building a model of the therapeutic process cross-culturally.

In part because of these findings, a common criticism applied to psychotherapy by its medical critics is that it is merely a dressed-up placebo. Placebo responses are the improvement in symptoms produced by supposedly nonactive substances (e.g., sterile water or a sugar pill). They are believed to work through the activation of physiological processes owing to the patient's faith in the treatment or the healer (Shapiro 1959). Placebos occupy a strange position in medicine (Brody 1977). Though they average a 35 percent improvement rate for medical conditions across the board, they are viewed by clinical researchers as a source of confounding effects in clinical trials of the efficacy of new treatment agents. In fact, placebo responses vary between 10 and 90 percent in such trials, and seem to be strongly influenced by the quality of the doctor-patient relationship (Moerman 1979). Rather than laud a powerful nonspecific treatment effect that all physicians should be trained to maximize, placebos are disdained by medical researchers and teachers.

Psychotherapy may very well be a way of maximizing placebo responses, a nonspecific treatment effect, but if so, it should be applauded, rather than condemned, for exploiting a useful therapeutic process which is underutilized in general health care. The placebo effect can be reconfigured as the activation through the process of interpersonal communication of a powerful endogenous therapeutic system that is part of the psychophysiology of all individuals and the sociophysiology of relationships (Hahn and Kleinman 1983)—what Lionel Tiger (1979) has called the biology of optimism. The comparison of psychotherapy to placebos also indicates the ambivalence with which medical science looks upon this archaic remnant of medicine's past. Psychotherapy is threatening to academics attempting to forge a psychiatric science because of its ties with folk and popular therapies and its "soft," psychosocial image. It is of great interest to the anthropologist, however, since it enables her to detect the fault lines that split the psychiatric profession into different camps.

Cross-cultural studies bring a broader perspective to the study of how the psychiatrist heals. Whereas the systems of psychotherapy constitute culturally salient psychiatric treatment in the West, they are not what the vast majority of non-Western psychiatrists do. The latter are engaged in very limited contact with large numbers of patients (usually five to fifteen minutes per patient), many with the most serious of disorders and some with the psychological effects of infectious diseases (i.e., depression, anxiety, cognitive deficit, withdrawal), a situation in which somatic therapies and a more medical approach are appropriate. Nonetheless, even in the Third World, psychiatrists do engage in brief supportive talk therapies not all that dissimilar from the preferred psychosocial treatment method of primary care physicians in the West. Attraction to psychotherapy is increasing in a number of non-Western societies, especially owing to the rapidly growing educated urban middle class familiar with Western ideas and strongly influenced by the world economic order which reproduces Western cultural forms, including psychological therapies, as commodities for consumption by this new elite class.

When I began my field research in Taiwan in 1968, there was hardly any psychotherapy available and little popular understanding of its uses. In the 1970s, the works of Freud and other key figures in psychological healing were translated into Chinese and published in Taiwan for an ever-expanding audience of students, professionals, and intellectuals generally. During this same period, Yang Kuo-shu (1986), an outstanding Taiwanese psychologist, demonstrated that the value orientation of college students was turning in a Western direction while maintaining many traditional values. Most notably, psychological-mindedness and individualism were on the increase. Not surprisingly, in recent years more clients have sought out psychotherapy, and it has become more prominent, though still nowhere near the North American level of popularity.

Much the same phenomenon is in a very early stage of development in China. During the last several years, the political liberalization in the mainland has witnessed the publication of scores of books on normal and abnormal psychology. Books which have printing runs of 10,000 to 30,000 copies are sometimes sold out the day they appear in the book stores. There is even a group of psychiatrists in Beijing who have introduced psychoanalytic psychotherapy, a method that was anathematized in the 1950s and attacked with great ferocity during the Cultural Revolution. Cognitive, behavioral, and supportive forms of psychotherapy are being introduced in China's major centers of psychiatric research and teaching. Psychiatrists in the developing countries have also been experimenting with the use of indigenous forms of healing which patients find more culturally acceptable. *Yoga* in India and *qi gong* in China are examples of indigenous practices widely available in psychiatric centers. The presence in those societies of active folk healing traditions—no longer enchanting to intellectuals raised with a secular vision—doubtless has contributed to the growth of interest in psychotherapy, and has also offered a model for *indigenizing* psychotherapy (Kapur et al. 1979; Kakar 1982).

Anthropologists, for good reason, are uncomfortable with the tendency of mental health professionals to elevate the Western paradigm of psychotherapy into a comparative grid that can be used to study indigenous healing systems worldwide. Rather, for the anthropologist, psychotherapy is merely one indigenous form of symbolic healing, i.e., a therapy based on words, myth, and ritual use of symbols (see Lévi-Strauss 1967; Turner 1967). The question of how the psychiatrist heals, then, becomes a question of comparing psychotherapy (along with the psychiatrist's other therapeutic practices) to a wide assortment of indigenous healing systems in non-Western societies, among traditionally oriented ethnic groups in Western society, and in the Western historical tradition. By demanding that psychotherapy be analyzed within this broader framework, thereby standing the ethnocentric mental health approach on its head, anthropologists seek to derive a comparative grid for studying the different forms of symbolic healing that is more scientifically valid for ascertaining cross-cultural universals in the healing process. Such a grid should also be sensitive to what is unique in each local healing system. Psychotherapy—what is it, what does it share with other healing systems, what are its effects, and how are they produced?—for the student of the world's cultures, is the question, not the solution.

In this chapter, I first compare psychotherapy (and other aspects of the psychiatrist's treatment) to healing systems in non-Western cultures and to other indigenous systems in the West, in order to demonstrate, in spite of the great diversity of "schools," that there are certain commonalities that can be discerned in cross-cultural perspective. What do these commonalities tell us about the structure of psychiatrist-patient relationships and the cultural influences on the ideology and process of psychotherapy? How does the psychotherapy practiced by psychiatrists, and indeed by all psychotherapists, produce its effects? Is there a method for translating psychotherapy into culturally relevant practice in radically different societies? What, then, is universal, what culture-specific, in the healing process?

A Comparative Cross-Cultural Grid for Assessing Psychotherapy as an Indigenous Healing System

When I review the cross-cultural literature on healing systems together with my own empirical research, juxtaposing shamans, other religious healers, doctors of traditional Chinese and Indian medicine, and the myriad of alternative practitioners and physicians of biomedicine, criteria emerge for comparing healing systems:[2]

(1) *Institutional Setting,* i.e., the specific location of the practitioners of a local healing system in a particular society's *folk, popular,* and *professional* arenas of care

(2) *Characteristics of the Interpersonal Interaction*
   (a) Number of participants
   (b) Time coordinates (i.e., episodic or continuous; length of time of interactions; etc.)
   (c) Quality of the relationships (i.e., formal or informal; authoritarian or egalitarian; degree of trust, warmth, support; etc.)
   (d) Attitudes of the participants toward each other.

(3) *Characteristics of the Practitioner*
   (a) Personality (charismatic, empathetic, disordered, etc.)
   (b) Reasons for becoming a healer
   (c) Rites of passage
   (d) Training
   (e) Career trajectory and clinical experience
   (f) Type of practice (including special interests and skills)
   (g) Status in the healing system and in community
   (h) Insight into the clinical process
   (i) Rewards and difficulties

(4) *Idioms of Communication*
   (a) Mode (i.e., somatic, religious, moral, psychological, social)
   (b) Code (i.e., nonverbal, verbal, special semiotic system)
   (c) Explanatory models of a particular illness episode (i.e., shared, conflicting, open, tacit, etc.)
   (d) Rhetorical devices for narratizing illness and negotiating treatment
   (e) Work of interpretation

(5) *Clinical Reality*
   (a) Sacred or secular
   (b) Disease-oriented/illness-oriented
   (c) Focus of treatment (i.e., patient, family, other)
   (d) Primary/secondary/tertiary level of medical system
   (e) Symbolic and/or instrumental interventions
   (f) Interrogative or open-ended
   (g) Patient-centered or practitioner-centered
   (h) Therapeutic expectations (including clients' emotional arousal and hope and therapists' belief in or need to prove self-efficacy)
   (i) Perceived locus of responsibility for care
   (j) Confession and moral witnessing

(6) *Therapeutic Stages and Mechanisms*
   (a) Process

(b) Mechanisms of change (i.e., catharsis, social learning and conditioning, persuasion, behavioral control, altered state of consciousness, sense of mastery, insight, etc.)
(c) Adherence
(d) Termination
(e) Evaluation of outcome (including toxicity and iatrogenesis)
(7) *Extratherapeutic Aspects*
(a) Social control
(b) Ethical codes and problems
(c) Economic costs and constraints on access
(d) Political implications

If we employ this grid to compare psychiatric care and specifically the most common form of psychotherapy practiced by psychiatrists in North America—a psychodynamically based method—with other symbolic healing systems (e.g., shamanism, other forms of religious healing, the literate Asian systems of traditional medicine, a variety of lay psychotherapies), then we quickly discover that the psychiatrist's care is unusual in a number of important ways.

To begin with, psychiatry has a peculiar relationship to the greater health care system and to its parent profession, biomedicine. Most symbolic healing around the globe occurs in the *popular* (family and community) and *folk* (nonbureaucratized and nonprofessionalized) sectors of care, not in *professional* institutions. Other, nonbiomedical professions of healing, such as osteopathy, chiropractic, naturopathy, Ayurveda (India's indigenous profession of medicine), traditional Chinese medicine, and professionalized indigenous healing systems in Japan, Thailand, and Pakistan emphasize symbolic healing to a greater degree than does biomedicine. Unlike biomedicine, they do not possess a psychiatric or other specialty for providing symbolic healing. That is the responsibility of each professional. In fact, there is some evidence to suggest that biomedicine as practiced in Asia and perhaps other non-Western settings is so strongly influenced by their indigenous models that it incorporates certain of these core symbols as part of the therapeutic skills of every physician; e.g., biomedical physicians in China often take the pulse in the style of Chinese medicine practitioners and inquire about aspects of diet that reflect concern for *yin/yang* balance (cf. Kleinman 1980; Weisberg 1984; Lock 1980). Perhaps one of psychiatry's latent functions is to legitimate a more substantial form of symbolic healing in biomedicine which makes the biomedical profession less unlike all the other healing systems by incorporating key symbolic forms of healing from the popular and folk healing sectors of the Western cultural tradition. This makes psychiatry distinctive from the rest of the profession of biomedicine, though more like other healing professions.

Psychiatric care, and biomedical care generally, as practiced in the

West, differs from other healing systems inasmuch as other systems of symbolic healing are not dyadic (they usually involve family members and friends) or private (they occur in public in the presence of family and other patients). Nor is most healing long-term, divorced from everyday life encounters between the participants, psychologically minded, secular, or oriented to the needs and rights of the individual as against those of the family and community. Only healing systems in the West are moving toward egalitarian models of the therapeutic relationship and a concept of open practitioner-client negotiations. Virtually all others emphasize authoritarian models and tacit (if any) negotiations. Non-Western healing systems, apart perhaps from Buddhist ones, usually do not regard insight as a necessary ingredient of therapeutic change, nor are individuation or personal growth explicit treatment goals. These contrasts illumine the radical differences between egocentric Western culture and sociocentric non-Western cultures, and disclose that culture exerts a powerful effect on care.

Psychiatric care is not unusual, however, in its pragmatic integration of somatic and symbolic treatment modalities. Many indigenous healing systems employ the laying on of hands, manipulation of the body, and the use of diet, drugs, exercise, and meditative techniques side by side with practical advice and symbolic rituals. Trust, empathy, and various other components of support, furthermore, are ubiquitous in healing everywhere. There are other, nontrivial cross-cultural similarities. Both psychotherapy and indigenous non-Western therapies encourage congruence in the explanatory models of patients and practitioners regarding the cause and nature of the disorder and in therapeutic expectations about what constitutes improvement. Mutually ambivalent attitudes of healers and clients are commonplace. Healers view patients as offering an opportunity for demonstrating their therapeutic powers (with all that connotes in prestige and reward) but also see them as a potential threat of negative outcomes, including failure. Medical-legal suits may be decidedly uncommon outside the West, but healers in a number of societies are expected to pay an indemnity if their patients die. In Taiwan, if the patient dies and the family believes the physician responsible, they sometimes may place the coffin in the practitioner's office until he offers a suitable financial compensation (Kleinman 1980). For shamans in South American Indian groups, death of the patient sometimes meant that their community would take their lives. Patients and their circles often view healers as the source or conduit of great powers for good, and simultaneously as self-interested parties who can do harm. This ambivalence is most striking in those societies where healers are also feared as sorcerers who can inflict illness.

This is not the place to analyze in detail the characteristics of practitioners; yet such a comparison would demonstrate again key cross-cultural similarities and differences, in the selection, training, career trajectory, clinical experience, status, and rewards and difficulties of practitioners—similarities and differences that reflect major cultural, political, economic, and institutional constraints on healers. One cross-cultural characteristic of healers is worthy of note: namely, personality. While there is little empirical evidence to confirm the hypothesis that healers are mentally ill, as an earlier generation of anthropologists speculated (Boyer 1974; Sasaki 1969; Opler, ed., 1959), there is support for the view that the more successful indigenous healers in the non-Western world may possess charismatic personalities that radiate power, inspire confidence, and demonstrate empathy for the patient's experience (Lambo 1974; Dean and Thong 1972; Eliade 1964; Handelman 1967; Harner, ed., 1973; Kleinman 1980; Taussig 1987; Turner 1967). Research on psychotherapists in North America repeatedly discloses the importance of the therapist's personality for therapeutic effects, and the tendency of effective therapists to have warm, supportive personalities (Truax and Carkhoff 1962; Strupp and Hadley 1979; Parloff et al. 1978; Luborsky et al., 1985). There is also an impression that successful healers may have a deeply personal need, intensified or even created by the social context, to be effective in the lives of others (Kleinman 1980, 1986). They need to believe in themselves and in the efficacy of their craft. A challenge to their sense of technical competence is a threat to their personal confidence. They feel inner pressure to succeed. I am not familiar with research on this subject that pertains to psychiatrists or psychotherapists generally, but it is my clinical experience that the psychiatrist's felt need to make his patients feel better is no less important an aspect of the psychiatrist's clinical success than it is of the shaman's. Perhaps this is an inner ingredient of successful practitioners of a wide range of types.

The mode of clinical communication between healer and client may be somatic, psychological, moral, religious, or social idioms of distress and care; their semiotic codes create a keyboard of nonverbal, verbal, and special signs through which these idioms are transmitted and received. For example, shamans in Taiwan use the language of gods, ghosts, or ancestors afflicting (or protecting) their clients to convey, in a culturally authorized idiom, not only practical religious concerns in the family's life but also key interpersonal tensions (Kleinman 1980). Thus, a remarkably insightful Taiwanese shaman whom I observed interpreted the acute back pain experienced by almost all the members of a family who had recently experienced the death, under highly questionable circumstances, of a young daughter-in-law as her unappeased ghost holding tightly to the backs of her intimate relatives in a display of righteous anger over the family turmoil which provoked her "suicide." The god possessing the shaman was the first to publically voice this menacing term, the expression of which, as the centerpiece of a culturally prescribed exorcism of the attacking ghost, quite literally authorized the outpouring of deeply ambivalent grief as well as something akin to penance and absolution. Csordas (1987) gives other examples from a Brazilian religious cult of a subtle interweaving of religious, psychological, and medical rhetorics of healing. Primary care practitioners worldwide are becoming aware that physical symptoms often represent bodily metaphors of complaints for negotiating personal and social troubles that, for one reason or another, cannot be dealt with openly (Katon et al. 1982). The patient complains of headaches and thereby conveys pain in the temples *and* a painful mental conflict to whose intensification or amelioration the medical care will contribute. It is estimated that between one-third and two-thirds of all visits to primary care practitioners may involve such negotiation of the central, if disguised, reason for care (Katon et al. 1984).

Patients, their family members, and healers differ significantly with respect to the rhetorical devices they employ to express and negotiate problems. Symptoms may be dramatically enacted in one cultural context and understated in another. Possession states (of patients and shamans) sanction powerful divine and demonic voices to demand redress or to insist on a therapeutic compromise (Lewis 1971). Individuals also differ, of course, in their talents for using culturally approved rhetorical techniques. Some are extremely effective at eliciting empathy or access to resources, others much less so. Some are spectacularly ineffective. The last include so-called chronic complainers worldwide, who in psychiatric care are labeled hysterics or hypochondriacs.

Interpretation is not by any means unique to psychoanalytic psychotherapy. It is a core task of healing cross-culturally. The practitioner must reconfigure the patient's illness narrative, within his therapeutic system's taxonomy, as a disease with a particular cause, understandable pathophysiology, and expectable course. Shamans as well as herbalists, faith healers as well as internists, *curanderos* (Mexican American folkhealers) and *espiritistas* (Puerto Rican spiritual healers) as well as psychotherapists must interpret somatic complaints as bodily icons of troubles in life's various domains (home, work place, school, street, interstices of the self). Nor is psychoanalysis the only healing system that elaborates an indigenous structure of exegesis for interpreting body symbols. The Ayurvedic practitioner in Bombay, the physician of traditional East Asian medicine in Kyoto, the Unani doctor in Karachi—all follow sophisticated native ethnotheories for understanding both *what* a particular episode of illness means and *how* illnesses' meanings are to be interpreted. The healing systems of different cultures and ethnic groups differ greatly, of course, with respect to the answers provided to these questions.

Healers and patients create a local ethos of expectations about clinical etiquette, action, and outcome that I have referred to as *clinical reality*. Psychotherapy's clinical reality as an aspect of psychiatric care is secular, disease- and illness-oriented, open-ended, usually more patient- than practitioner-centered, and often involves an eclectic mix of symbolic and instrumental interventions. Expectations of successful outcome tend to be more long-term and modest than in acute medical care; the perceived locus of control is the sick person; and care frequently invokes, though psychiatrists may not recognize it as such, a kind of moral witnessing of the patient's life with some degree of confession of difficulties usually kept from others. Generalization is difficult, because different psychotherapies vary on all these axes. Psychotherapeutic systems also diverge over whether the function of therapy is seen as improving the patient's adaptation to society or criticizing societal demands and motivating the patient toward social reform by projecting his individual problems outward onto the social structure and encouraging practical engagement in social change, or at least individual fortitude and courage to assert himself in the face of the social system. Most forms of psychotherapy tend toward the conservative (maintain the status quo) end of this spectrum, but various radical therapies encourage reform and even revolt.

Non-Western healing systems have greatly different clinical realities: often they emphasize sacred reality, illness orientation (meaning that they take the patient's account of the problem as their central concern), symbolic intervention, interrogative structure, family-centered locus of control (there may even be a family or lay therapy management team which makes the crucial decisions in care—see Janzen 1978), and substantial expectations of change, even cure. Like Western systems they differ greatly as to whether they serve conservative or reformist interests. Confession and moral witnessing are central to some non-Western systems, peripheral or even absent in others.

Most therapeutic systems world-wide appear to create emotional arousal in clients and to stimulate the feeling of hope. Even if they don't explicitly aim to remoralize clients and family members, that is often their effect. To do this, it has been argued, the healer must believe in his therapy (Torrey 1986).

Of course, conventional biomedicine also differs from psychiatric care on a number of these axes. It tends to be oriented to disease (the pathology held to underlie the patient's complaints), instrumental interventions, interrogation, and a practitioner-centered version of clinical reality. Emotional arousal of patients, encouragement of hope and faith in the treatment, and remoralization of patients and family members are aspects of effective biomedical care too. It can be argued, however, that its intensive preoccupation with technology and with the formal logic of clinical decision making gives medical students the dangerous message that the emotional response of the patient and the practitioner's own personal investment in the treatment matter much less than the technology applied and the rationale for its use. This is a sign of the marginal status of psychiatric concerns within the profession of medicine.

All forms of healing create conditions for catharsis, though some are much more effective than others at eliciting this important therapeutic process. Where the therapeutic ethos encourages the patient's attachment to healing symbols that are neither too remote from nor too close to the patient's emotional experience, catharsis is more likely to occur (Scheff 1983). Psychotherapies obviously differ in their cathartic efficacy, but on the whole, catharsis is much more important to psychiatric care than it is to other forms of biomedical treatment. Catharsis is a therapeutic process in most non-Western symbolic healing systems. Psychophysiological change and social persuasion are also nearly universal. So commonly do these therapeutic elements, along with the previously mentioned expectant faith in a positive outcome and shared world view of healer and patient, occur together that Frank (1974) and Pentony (1981) advance comparative models of healing cross-culturally in which social persuasion, made possible by shared beliefs and expectations, intensifies expectant faith which in turn contributes to catharsis and psychophysiological change. They considered these to be the central elements in all therapeutic effects. While emphasizing different components, Torrey (1986) and Karasu (1986) claim that it is these kinds of things that make healing effective.

Havens's (1985) important insight into the role of irony, paradox, and other rhetorical devices that can break through the conventions of mundane discourse in psychotherapy to foster therapeutic alliance may seem to some so clearly characteristics of the contemporary Western tradition that they are sure to be candidates for a unique therapeutic process in symbolic healing. But in fact this is not the case. Many indigenous healing traditions—e.g., Zen-based therapies in Japan (Reynolds 1983) and South American Indian shamans who use hallucinogens (Harner, ed., 1973)—apparently make use of these tropes for some of the same reasons Havens recommends: to make contact with nonrational aspects of the self and to promote emotional change. This is not how they are conceptualized by those who apply them in the hurly-burly of clinical work, yet this is what serious students of the subject have come to believe (Leighton et al. 1968; Reynolds 1976; Kapur et al. 1979; Kakar 1982).

Ethnographic accounts of healing rituals in non-Western societies—e.g., Turner's (1967) writings on Ndembu healing; Janzen's (1978) description of the Bakongo; Fabrega and Silver's (1973) discussion of shamanistic healing in Zinacantan; and Tambiah's (1977) account of Buddhist healing in Thailand—point to the universality of a tripartite process. In the first movement, an underlying casual agent is announced (e.g., the ghost clinging to the backs of bereaved family members). It is affirmed in the healing system's authorized taxonomy, and then established as a particular instance of the generalized interpretive structure that stands behind the system (e.g., the idea among traditionally oriented Taiwanese that the "hungry" ghosts of daughters-in-law who suicide because they are wronged can plague a family with illness and other misfortunes until they are ritually propitiated). In the second phase, the symbolic form that causes or materializes pathology (in this instance, the ghost) is manipulated via therapeutic rituals (sacred or secular). Finally, the causal agent, on the plane of the interpretive system's core symbols, is removed (i.e., the ghost is exorcised and the shaman ceremonially pronounces its departure); the healing is affirmed, performatively, since it meets the authorized criteria, to be successful: the ritual of exorcism, if appropriately chosen and properly enacted, is said to work. A new symbolic status—cured, improved, "feelin' better," or, in our example, free of ghost and protected against its return—is announced and consecrated. Psychiatric care—including psychodynamic psychotherapy's early (the neurotic problem is recognized as having been caused by an Oedipal conflict), middle (the conflict is worked through), and termination (the patient is helped to believe that the neurotic conflict is understood and resolved) periods—shares this processual structure with an odd assortment of bedfellows, including Northwest Coast Indian healing ceremonies (Jilek 1982), charismatic Catholic healing (Csordas 1984), traditional Chinese medicine (Kleinman 1980), the therapeutic rites of Kung Bushmen (Katz 1982), *yoga* (Neki 1974), Puerto Rican spiritism (Harwood 1977), and Haitian voodoo (Metraux 1959).

Psychoanalytic psychotherapy's emphatic endorsement of change in the core personality of the sick individual, isolated from kin and social circle; its preoccupation with uncovering unconscious conflicts within the deep interiority of the mind that are hidden by defenses that originate in early childhood and that, once effectively understood, can be mastered; and its identification of central conflicts almost entirely with sexual drives—all have been shown to derive from special themes in the Western cultural tradition (Rycroft 1986). There are few non-Western analogues. But we can point to phenomena like trust, empathy, moral witnessing, and the other elements of support—practical problem solving, clarification, explanation, and a variety of rhetorical devices (like nonverbal and verbal signs that the therapist believes in the patient's sense of mastery) used to remoralize and persuade—that are by no means peculiar to the Western tradition and its cultural modes of healing (Frank 1974; Leighton et al. 1968; Murphy 1964; Harwood 1977; Reynolds 1976; Csordas 1984).

Many observers of healing ritual have posited psychophysiological effects of autonomic nervous system arousal and psychoneuroimmunological and endocrinological activation (Prince, ed., 1982). But convincing evidence of the effect of therapeutic rituals on the secretion of endogenous opiates (which in theory should raise pain thresholds and damp the disabling effects of painful symptoms) and other neurohumoral agents (e.g., the brain's neurotransmitters) has not been published. Nonetheless, hardly any serious students of healing rituals doubt that significant biological effects result from catharsis, conditioning, and the other mechanisms of therapeutic change. Most psychiatrists believe that one or more of the same processes underwrite potentially powerful biological effects in psycho-therapy.

Altered states of consciousness (e.g., trance and possession), on the sur-face, would appear to be an interesting source of differences between psychiatry and indigenous folk healing systems. Among members of non-Western groups and of traditionally oriented ethnic minorities and reli-gious groups in the West with intact faith healing traditions, states of trance and possession are commonplace. They quite clearly are associated with potentially profound psychophysiological changes. Prior to the mod-ern era of Western history, these altered states were ubiquitous in folk and popular healing traditions in the West too. But they are not widely found among middle-class Westerners in contemporary society. Nor does psychi-atry or the rest of modern biomedicine seem to employ techniques for in-ducing possession. Yet, in fact, meditation and a wide assortment of tech-niques to induce relaxation (including hypnosis) are used by physicians, albeit to alter the consciousness of patients not healers. Meditation clearly brings about an alteration in state of consciousness. Technically, hypnosis, still popular in psychiatry, is controlled trance. Thus, in the disenchanted modern West, meditation, hypnosis, and other relaxation techniques ap-pear to have replaced possession states as the major lay and professional forms for enlisting altered states of consciousness in the service of therapeu-tic change. Again a cross-cultural universal in the healing process connects psychiatry with healing traditions in other societies, with those who prac-tice sacred folk healing in the West, and with historical traditions.

Termination is a notoriously significant issue in psychotherapy; it is less robust though still an issue in other healing systems. Adherence to pre-scribed treatments and proscribed activities turns out to be problematic in folk healing and self-care as well as professional therapies (cf. Chrisman n.d.), but it is "hypocognized"—not raised to the status of a self-conscious question—in virtually all other systems than biomedical care. Transfer-ence and countertransference can be shown to occur in many types of treat-ment, but their explicit analysis is unique to psychoanalytic psychother-apy. These two concepts may represent the most important contribution of psychotherapy to the cross-cultural comparison of healing systems.

The power of clinical reality can extend beyond the practitioner-patient relationship to the larger social arena. Movements of social change—re-form, revolution, and reactionary revanchism—have not infrequently en-hanced their legitimacy by invoking therapeutic metaphors. For example, the major rebellions in China in the Han dynasty, in the much more recent Qing dynasty, and in the twentieth century either grew out of healing movements or used the imagery of curing China's political sicknesses (Dull 1975). The Chinese Communist revolution played up the idea of curing the "sick man of Asia." The Nazis expropriated the metaphor of healing in their ideological defense of the need to extirpate "the rotten appendix of the Jews" in the Aryan body. Lifton (1986) demonstrates how, in medicine's most evil hour, healing came to quite literally mean killing for the Nazi concentration camp doctors.

Social control (*pace* the antipsychiatrists, who would have us believe it is a creation of either psychiatry or the modern state) is an inalienable aspect of healing in every society. Indeed, if anything, the social control aspects of healing systems are greater in non-Western societies (Cawte 1974). That is to say, sickness as a social phenomenon presents the members of the social system with two challenging questions: bafflement ("Why me?") and control ("What to do?"). Sickness is a threat to the social order—in the forms of epidemic disorders, incapacitating disability, and severe mental illness, literally so. The ordering of symptoms into illness is an initial step in a process that goes on to involve various levels of control—personal, familial, network, institutional, community, societal. Control is exerted through the application of technical interventions and social authority. The occasion to exercise control may be an illness episode and the social tensions it either results from or exacerbates, but control can be, and often is, extended beyond healing to social relations generally.

Think of the frequently intrusive surveillance of families by child mental health authorities in North America who, through consultation in school or health clinic, have detected a significant behavioral problem. The original problem—enuresis, anorexia, hyperactivity, antisocial behavior—leads to referral of the whole family for evaluation. That evaluation, and the recommendation for family counseling that often results, may well have therapeutic significance. But it also is a form of control extended from the child to the entire family, who are told directly or by implication that they may well be the source of the difficulty. They are "followed" with assessment schedules, formal interviews, and measures of family functioning that will establish whether they are "normal," or "deviant," or "at risk." All of this observation, counseling, and recording is conducted in a language of medical problems and their treatment. Yet the effect of focusing attention on the family, intended or unintended, is to alert its members that they may be at fault and should change their ways. Whatever else it is, this is the diffusion of control into the nuclear social unit (cf. Lasch 1977; Donzelot 1980; Castel et al. 1982). Much the same happens with child and adolescent psychiatric disorders, and especially following allegations of child or spouse abuse. As interest in therapeutic and preventive family interventions intensifies, we can expect a much wider array of disorders to trigger these forays of health and mental health experts into the home.

On several occasions, psychiatric colleagues of mine from China have been surprised both by the propensity of North American health experts to enter into families to "protect" children and the willingness of courts to make rulings about what *should* happen in the home, including what is to many Chinese an astounding misuse of legal authority, the court's willingness to remove children from the custody of their parents. They note that in their "totalitarian" society, the home is not regarded as an appropriate sphere of medical or legal intervention. Of course, China's block associations, building committees, and informal oversight over personal behavior in the work unit look to North American eyes like an even more intrusive social system.

In small-scale preliterate societies like the Kung Bushmen or Mbuti Pygmies, healing involves the entire community. There are no specialists to impose authority; rather, it emerges within the community consensus. In tribal and peasant societies, accusations of witchcraft and sorcery as the cause of illness may lead to trials, punishment, and ostracism. In large-scale, industrial societies, social control of sickness is exerted by a variety of sources—the courts, community welfare and law enforcement agencies, the healing professions, ultimately the national government. The psychiatrist, like other health professionals, may be informally expected or formally charged by the laws of the state to undertake certain forms of control. In recent decades in industrialized societies, and now in the most rapidly modernizing nonindustrialized societies as well, as I discussed in Chapters 4 and 5, social problems are medicalized, transformed from moral or legal into therapeutic questions. Psychiatry in many societies has led the way in this process, not because of the policies of the profession, but because of those of the society. We have every reason to suspect that certain of the misuses of psychiatry in the West also exist, though perhaps to a lesser extent, in the non-Western world. This is as important a question for future cross-cultural research as is its corollary: protection of the rights of psychiatric patients, including those treated in psychotherapy. There may be fewer abuses of psychiatric care in the non-Western world, but there is also less protection of patient's rights. For example, in familistic societies, patients can be hospitalized involuntarily through the connivance of their families and their psychiatrists. Most therapeutic agencies in the Third World offer no protection of confidentiality. The patient's problems are exposed in public and not always to a supportive audience. Even indigenous healing systems may coerce, threaten, and abandon patients. Charlatans and quacks are to be found in all healing systems, preying on the desperate and powerless. Finally, there is excessive use of ECT, because patients in Third World psychiatry usually have little input into professional decision making. While ethical codes of behavior for professional psychotherapists in the West have been at times self-serving, often have not been effectively enforced, and do not cover lay therapists, in much of the developing world there are no formal codes at all for holding healers accountable.

Another ethical (and legal) question that is quite central to the discussion of healing is how to assure that healers are competent, and that patients are protected from those who are not. In his race along the broadest possible avenues of agreement among selected cross-cultural studies of healers, which aims to arrive at simple universals in the psychotherapeutic process, while trying not to lose his way in the maze of winding, narrow back streets of detail that illumine even more extensive cultural differences, Fuller Torrey (1986), a psychiatrist writing for a popular audience, offers an answer to this question. Let us establish, says Torrey, local regulations for licensing and standards for practice for all healers—psychotherapists and witchdoctors. The suggestion is as seductively simplistic as the rest of Torrey's survey. It is a solution geared to a professional sector of practice where schools, exams, licensing formalities, standards of practice, and formal ethical codes are to be found as part of the bureaucratic structure of health care. In such a system—such as professional psychotherapy in North America—such a recommendation would have a good chance to be successful. And I too would support it.

But folk healers do not practice in professional institutions. The folk healing sector of care by definition is greatly pluralistic, unlicensed, unregulated, and at its ambiguous margins quasi-legal or even illegal. Passing regulations and standards for folk healers will almost certainly accomplish several undesirable things in Benin as well as Bogotá, Benares, and Boston. First, folk healers will be professionalized. Or rather those most like professional practitioners will be coopted into the professional system, usually under the control of professional practitioners. A psychiatrist from Sumatra once told me that he wanted all the folk healers in his region enumerated and licensed so that he could determine who would be allowed to practice, and those selected would then practice under his direction. "I can see at most 100 patients a day on my own." But he said, rubbing his hands in anticipation of the financial reward, "If I employed ten folk healers, I could see 1000 patients!" One can well imagine the abuses that would result. In addition, professionalizing folk healing may attenuate or routinize just those practices that are most central to its success: empathy, sacred authority, trial-and-error innovation within tradition, minimal objectification of personal problems, and nonroutinization of practice.

Second, regulations will drive many folk healers underground, criminalizing practices that are already at the margins of legality. There is some empirical evidence from urban Africa that when folk healers are barred or severely controlled, predatory practices intensify, real criminals begin to see folk healing as a way of bilking the public, and laymen go to lengths to circumvent official obstacles in the search for care.

Torrey's temptation, as I shall call it, to bureaucratize practice and extend professional authority over the training and surveillance of practitioners is appropriate for pastoral counselors and the wide range of alternative professional or paraprofessional therapists in North America, who should be held to the same standards for psychotherapy as psychiatrists, psychologists, and social workers. But it is a prescription for creating disaster in folk healing circles. Rather, folk healers should be brought under closer supervision of local communities, not professional organizations, and that control should be loose enough to allow a wide variety of practitioners to flourish as long as there is no evidence of actually dangerous, unethical, or illegal practices.

Economic costs of psychotherapy and constraints on access, which in the past have contributed to the formation of a largely middle-class clientele, are significant issues for current policy debate (see McGrath and Lowson 1986; Goleman 1985b). Insofar as psychotherapy has been found cost-effective in reducing so-called overutilization of primary care services and hospitalizations and in treating the common psychiatric conditions depression and anxiety as well as so-called "life problems"—e.g., marital conflicts, midlife crises, adolescent turmoil (see Mumford et al. 1984; Bloch and Lambert 1985; Borus et al. 1985)—the next-level question of cost effectiveness must turn on the findings that successful outcome does not seem to depend on the type or extent of the therapist's training. The logical argument would seem to be that if psychiatrists in the U.S. doing psychotherapy charge, say $75 to $100 per session, psychologists $50 to $75, social workers $35 to $50, and paraprofessionals even less, and all have the same outcome, why, then, what rationale can there be for governmental or third-party insurers paying for anything above the minimum? To forestall this coming query, psychiatrists, psychologists, and social workers actively lobby to protect their share of a market which, as I have noted, is increasingly dominated by a plethora of types of lay therapists, about whose cost efficacy almost nothing is known. True, few if any of these lay practitioners and alternative professionals receive third-party reimbursement. Nevertheless, if we are to take the economics of psychotherapy seriously, these practitioners must be included in the calculations. And so too must be primary health care professionals—internists, family physicians, and nurse practitioners—who treat the "hidden psychiatric morbidity," namely about 60 percent of the mentally ill (Regier et al., 1978).

This is a greatly vexed issue. On the one hand, many patients seem willing to pay a great deal more than the minimum in order to secure access to higher-status professionals. Their conviction of the competence of their therapists may well play a role in the efficacy of the care they receive. On the other hand, access to all forms of health care in the U.S. has declined for the poor (Robert Wood Johnson Foundation 1987), who in the past have not been well served by psychotherapists of any kind. While the situation is particularly deplorable in the disorganized multitiered health system in the U.S., the place of psychotherapy in the British National Health Service and in other state-run health care systems is still being fought over (McGrath and Lowson 1986).

Indigenous healing systems in the non-Western world are not immune from these problems (Bannerman et al., eds., 1983). While certain traditional medicinal preparations, e.g., deer penis and bear claw in the pharmacopeia of Chinese medicine, and ritual practices, e.g., a nine-night Navaho sing, may be as expensive as or even more expensive than comparable biomedical treatment, it is my impression from what limited information has been published that many folk and popular health and mental health practices are affordable, if often just barely so, for rural and urban poor in developing societies. These same societies, however, provide very limited if any financial support for professional psychosocial services, and exclude most folk healing systems from reimbursement schemes. Thus, the burden of financing psychosocial care in many societies—north and south, east and west—falls squarely on the shoulders of individuals and families, perpetuating a long-standing problem of equity.

Heretofore, most research in this area has focused on macroeconomic aspects of psychotherapy and psychiatric care generally. What are now needed are microeconomic studies which tell us much more about the local determinants and consequences of lay decision making, help seeking and choice of healer in the lives of afflicted persons in need of care and their families.

Of all the extratherapeutic aspects of healing, its political implications are the most provocative. Taussig (1987) and Comaroff (1985), among others, argue that indigenous healing practices, such as shamanism among impoverished Indians in Columbia and native evangelical church healing among a Tswana group in South Africa, are forms of political resistance to colonial oppression and the ideology of the ruling class. Taussig, a physician-anthropologist, writes an entire book (1987) about shamanism in South America paying hardly any attention to what happens to the particular complaints of clients and thereby gives the astonishing impression that this indigenous form of clinical work may originate from attempts to deal with the symptoms of sick persons but really is about something altogether different:

> The power of the imagery brought to life by misfortune and its healing . . .
> is a power that springs into being where the life story is fitted as allegory to
> myths of conquest, savagery, and redemption. It should be clear by now
> that magic and religious faith involved in this are neither mystical nor prag-
> matic, and certainly not blind adherence to blinding doctrine. Instead, they
> constitute an imageric [sic] epistemology splicing certainty with doubt, and
> despair with hope, in which dreaming—in this case of poor country
> people—reworks the significance of imagery that ruling-class institutions
> such as the Church have appropriated for the task of colonizing utopian
> fantasies.

The radical analysis of this academic shaman—which at its most extreme would have us believe that biomedical practice among the impoverished in Colombia is worthless and even contributes to the powerlessness of the poor, while the shamans' hallucinogenic séances transcend the mundane mystifications of practical treatment for life-threatening infantile diarrhea and adult infections to offer an alternative political rhetoric of the oppressed—is so excessive as to be silly and, from a public health perspective, will be seen as an example of the dangerously romantic reverse ethnocentricism of wild anthropology.

And yet the serious student of healing will realize there is a kernel of truth buried in Taussig's overgrown tangle of deconstructionist tropes—one that receives far too little attention in the comparative cross-cultural literature on healing. Healing systems—professional as well as folk—can, though often they do not, offer interpretations that challenge orthodox political definitions of reality (e.g., Taiwanese shamanistic religious cults, in the past, offered one of the only permitted visible symbols of Taiwanese nationalism). They can contest the routinization of suffering and societal ideologies that seek to justify it. Folk healers as much as psychotherapists can revivify or instill personal and family hope through moral metaphors that contradict the corrosive self-images of an age that, like our own, seems obsessed with economic and biological determinist rhetorics of personal gain and narcissistic desire, and in their place reaffirm transcendence. And psychotherapists and other healers can reject clichéd soap-opera solutions to personal crises, which reinforce the politically expedient and commercially profitable illusion that we live in a domesticated "natural" world of expectable order in which disorder is atypical and need not be endured. In the place of this illusion, psychotherapists and other healers can offer the hard-won critical—and therefore moral as well as political—awareness that our experiences are difficult, uncertain struggles with menace and loss in local life worlds over which we exert imperfect control, sometimes hardly any, and in which the transformation of impending chaos into transient order is, for most of us, a precarious victory to be won (or lost) every day with usually inadequate resources and within an intimate circle of interdependence on others.

When healers reaffirm, as in my experience they more commonly do, the status quo and convert social predicaments into psychological conflicts and thereby blind us to the political roots of our all too human dilemmas (as D. M. Thomas's fictional Freud does in *The White Hotel* because his psychoanalysis of a hysterical German Jewish woman in Germany in the 1930s fails to take into account the social reality of Nazism and its personal effects on her life and his)—when we healers do this, then we must be reminded of the political antecedents and consequences of healing, which should be as routine a consideration in our self-reflective understanding of what our work is about as is the libidinal component of our countertransference. If Rudolph Virchow, who pioneered the study of both cellular pathology and social pathology in medicine, could say with the conviction of a revolutionary who manned the barricades in 1848, "Politics is nothing but medicine on a grand scale," perhaps we can reverse and appropriately moderate the saying to affirm that "healing is at times politics on a small scale."

Thus far, I have compared the psychiatrist's psychotherapy to folk healing without directly addressing the central question of comparative efficacy, or what such a comparison can tell us about how symbolic healing of any kind works. We know psychotherapy works, but what evidence do we have that folk healing is effective? Before we are entitled to use this comparison to illuminate the healing process, we surely must respond to this question. There is in fact evidence that at least some forms of folk healing are effective for certain kinds of disorders and interpersonal problems. First, it is essential to reemphasize that folk healing is not a single phenomenon, but a greatly heterogeneous set of practitioners and practices, running from legitimate, officially sanctioned healers to quasi-legal practitioners to outright charlatans and quacks (Snow 1978; Baer 1981; McGuire 1983). Substantial anecdotal evidence from ethnographers demonstrates that patients treated by folk healers generally feel better and members of the local social group generally believe them to be better. (Among hundreds of ethnographic observations of particular folk healing sessions, see Harwood 1977; Garrison 1977; Crapanzano 1973; Fabrega and Silver 1973; Lewis 1971; Turner 1967; Tambiah 1977; McGuire 1983; Nichter 1981; Kakar 1982; Eisenberg 1985; Good et al. 1982) Such encounters usually have not involved long-term follow-up or systematic assessment, however.

Systematic evaluations of the therapeutic outcomes of various folk healing approaches also disclose that local indigenous systems of symbolic healing have rates of successful outcome similar to those found in general medical care. Kleinman and Gale (1982), for example, compared 250 matched patients treated by folk healers and internists in Taiwan and discovered that more than 70 percent of patients treated by both types of practitioners improved. Kleinman and Song's (1979) earlier study of outcome of patients treated by Taiwanese shamans showed in a small sample that all felt better except those with acute severe medical problems. Finkler's (1983, 1985) study of patients treated by spiritist practitioners in rural Mexico documented high rates of success, especially for patients with somatized depression, anxiety, and life problems. Ness's study (1980) of a Pentecostal healing church in Newfoundland and Dobkin de Rios's (1981) research on a Peruvian healer came to similar conclusions, as have other studies reviewed in Csordas (1984). As a result of these and other empirical investigations, the WHO's review of indigenous healing (Bannerman et al., eds., 1983) recommended that health professionals learn to work together with selected types of folk healers in the Third World. Cross-cultural investigations have also documented definite limitations (see below) to this form of treatment as well as certain, not very common, toxicities—e.g., minor side effects of herbal remedies, advice that interferes with medical treatment, and feelings of guilt for not improving. But on the whole, most patients studied after visiting folk healers experience symptom relief, and a sense, usually shared by family members, that their conditions are improved.

More systematic outcome studies also indicate that many of the ecstatic claims for folk healing are grossly exaggerated, and that most success occurs in the treatment of self-limited acute conditions, in that of chronic disorders for which there is no cure, and in the management of psychosocial distress. Nonetheless, since these problems constitute the bulk of problems brought to primary care practitioners around the world, this is a significant accomplishment. Intriguingly, Kleinman and Gale (1982) discovered that both shamans and internists in Taiwan performed poorly in the treatment of patients with somatized psychiatric diseases, a finding that goes counter to the impression given by many students of this subject that folk healers are particularly effective in treating psychiatric disorders. Although these quantitative studies do indicate that folk healing can be effective, double-blind clinical trials have been impossible to conduct to determine which elements in indigenous healing practices are responsible for their efficacy. Thus, what follows is a summary of anthropological and cross-cultural psychiatric speculation on this topic.

How Psychotherapy and Other Forms of Symbolic Healing Heal?

A number of anthropologists have attempted to synthesize the leading cross-cultural theories and ethnographic data about symbolic healing into a model of how all symbolic healing works (cf. Douglas 1970; Dow 1986; Glick 1967; Horton 1967; Janzen 1978; Kleinman and Song 1979; Messing 1968; Moerman 1979; Nash 1967; Tambiah 1968; Turner 1967; Wallace 1959; and Young 1977). Their reviews provide a useful introduction for examining the process of psychotherapy from the vantage point of comparative research on how words and relationships create therapeutic effects. I shall first restate in my own terms a consensus model that emerges from the work of these and other scholars of symbolic healing; thereafter, I will draw on the materials and the ideas brought together in this model for a broader discussion of the place of psychiatric healing in contemporary health care. I hardly need to argue that psychotherapy makes a special contribution to medical care. I do wish to show that the processes underpinning how psychotherapy heals raise a troubling paradox at the heart of medicine.

Four structural processes appear to be essential to accomplish symbolic healing.

Stage I posits the presence of a *symbolic bridge* between personal experience, social relations, and cultural meanings that I have elaborated at several places in this book. The experiences of individuals in society (e.g., serious loss or misfortune) are signs whose meanings link up with a group's master symbols (e.g., *yin/yang*, the crucified Christ, or the body/self as a broken machine). Those symbols are the deep cultural grammar governing how the person orients himself to the world around him and to his inner world. That cultural grammar is found in the central myths (e.g., the Koran or the Constitution) that authorize the values of the group and that serve as a template for the personal myths of the individual. There is a hierarchy of linked systems running from cultural symbols to social relations and on to self and bodily processes. That hierarchy is the biopsychocultural basis for healing: it underwrites the "upward" assimilation of personal experience into cultural meanings and the "downward" particularization of those meanings into bodily processes via the cognition and affect of a particular person in a particular situation.

Sebeok (1986), a leader in semiotics, suggests these systems are evolutionarily linked through the development of codes for communicating at cellular, psychological, and behavioral levels. Genetic code, the neurotransmitter code, the code of endocrine hormones, and codes communicating meanings in social relations and cultural symbol systems—all are of very different types, but as communication systems are meaningfully interrelated (cf. Staiano 1986; Hofer 1984). That is to say, in human systems biological codes and codes of perception and behavior are made, through socialization processes, to relate, resonate, and even transact (cf. Werner and Kaplan 1967). Just as illness is projected at different levels of the biopsychocultural hierarchy (see Engel 1980), so too is healing a transformation of these recursive systems. For example, a Taiwanese healing ritual may remoralize a depressed young housewife by mobilizing husband, in-laws, and parents to offer emotional and practical support and by authorizing her special status in the community and time away from onerous duties in the home, because her symptoms are interpreted as evidence the gods have chosen her as a spirit medium. The ritual itself elicits catharsis, trance, and a powerful feeling of faith and hope. These, in turn, recruit autonomic nervous system, neuroendocrine, and limbic system reactions that reverse the physiology of depression. The first stage of symbolic healing, then, is the presence of the sociosomatic linkage. When lived experience in a shared community of meaning is not its source, initiation into a particular system of healing—e.g., charismatic Catholic prayer group or psychoanalytic relationship—is.

Stage II commences when this symbolic connection is activated for a particular person. A patient seeks out a healer. The healer persuades the patient that the problem from which he is suffering can be redefined in terms of the authorizing system of cultural meaning (i.e., hallucinations are the work of the devil and therefore can be treated by exorcism). In small-scale preliterate societies and in many developing societies as well, healer, patient, and family are usually in agreement about those core meanings (though as McCreery 1979 shows, this is not always the case.) The pluralism of large-scale, industrialized, secular societies is certainly different, yet an analogy can be drawn. For there still are some shared authorizing meanings, in spite of social fragmentation and personal disenchantment. Moreover, the healing system itself (think of psychoanalysis or behavioral therapy or a religious cult) involves specific professional or institutional symbol systems, in which patients are socialized. The healer interprets the patient's problem in the precise terms of these codes. But clearly more than interpretation takes place. The healer uses various rhetorical devices essential for social persuasion to convince the patient that the redefinition of the problem via the authorizing meaning system is valid. This is a reciprocal movement. Healer affirms and patient accepts; healer elicits trust and belief, and patient actively participates in the therapeutic ethos and commits himself to it, often passionately. The patient's experience comes to resonate with, or is conditioned by, the symbolic meanings of the healing system. The problem *and* the patient begin to be changed by the healer's redefinition of the situation, which involves a switching of communicative codes (e.g., from bodily pain to imbalance in *yin* and *yang*, or from melancholy to possessing demons or a childhood-based neurotic conflict).

In *Stage III* the healer skillfully guides therapeutic change in the patient's emotional reactions (which means bodily processes as well as self-processes) through mediating symbols that are particularized from the general meaning system. These are the symbols manipulated in healing rituals—e.g., the Navaho singer's images of the sacred mountains, his sand painting's figures of Navaho spirits, and the story that he sings. It is somewhat easier to see the psychotherapist's concrete clarifications and interpretations as symbols that are authorized, negotiated, and deeply felt in the psychotherapeutic sessions. It is not merely the healer's rhetorical skill at work here. The clinical reality of the healing interaction, constructed by the mutual expectations of the participants, contributes to the generalization of personal experience into therapeutic meaning system— e.g., the reinterpretation and re-experiencing of menacing amorphous demoralization as the specified anxiety of Oedipal conflict or the felt depression of blocked flow of energy—and the particularization of symbolic meaning into personal experience—e.g., from the family therapist's general idea of personal pathology representing hidden family conflicts to its concrete instantiation in an adolescent's experience of his overwhelming fear of parental divorce as the understandable and therefore treatable rage of delinquent acting out.

In *Stage IV*, the healer confirms the transformation of the particularized symbolic meaning—e.g., the invading spirit, now named, is subjected to specific rituals of exorcism, or the Oedipal conflict, now understood in the details of a personal history, is worked through in the interpretation of personal events and in the experience of its transference to the analyst. This symbolic transformation activates the dialectic linking culture (symbolic code) and social relations, on the one side, and psychobiology (autonomic nervous system and neuroendocrine system) on the other, to foster a desired (hoped for, believed in) change in the patient's emotions, disordered physiology, and social ties. In anthropological terms, the healing interaction fosters this transformation as a work of culture: the making over of psychophysiological process into meaningful experience and the affirmation of success.

Meanings mediate change at different levels of the hierarchy. The parallelism between symbolic world and body/self processes which was held to be the means by which healing restructures the person and the disorder may not be nearly as tight as students of ritual once claimed it to be (e.g., Lévi-Strauss 1969; Douglas 1970). The client may not be fully aware of the intricate meanings of the symbol system (Laderman 1986). Rather, it may be his early conditioning to key cultural codes—sounds, smells, words, images—that are now physiologically effective even if only partially or wrongly understood, or his placebo-like response to more general meanings of trust in the healer's competence and a conviction that the ritual, no matter the details, will make one better—it may be these things that constitute efficacy.

Healing, as a sacred or secular ritual, achieves its efficacy through the transformation of experience. That transformation is created out of the effective enactment of culturally authorized interpretations. Demons are exorcised, and the anxious patient comes to believe that the cause of the problem has been removed; that conviction, elicited by the therapeutic ethos and encouraged by the social circle, alters cognitive processes of hypervigilance and fearful appraisal of new situations to create a different emotional state: calm instead of apprehension and faith in mastery over life problems that previously were feared to be uncontrollable. What has changed? The life problems may or may not have been directly affected (i.e., the patient may still have to work under the same pressure imposed by his supervisor; or, on the other hand, owing to the attention a patient has received and the advice of the healer, an inattentive husband may become more supportive). How these problems are perceived, however, is no longer the same (e.g., a childhood trauma of rejection by a parent which has helped shape the patient's poor self-image and vulnerability to depression following the break-up of a close friendship, when it has been worked through in the transference and in grief work for the dead parent, is now not perceived as terrifying or responded to with intense guilt). Altered meanings exert practical efficacy in the felt experience of the patient, e.g., remoralizing the demoralized, and in the social tensions of the patient's circle, e.g., reconciling angry family members (Tambiah 1977; Kapferer 1983; Turner 1967).

Think of this change in terms of Scheff's (1979) model of catharsis. The healer encourages emotional distancing and release through the experiencing of mediating symbols. That emotional change alters the patient's cognitions (e.g., the intense envy and self-grandiosity that mask a deeply hurtful but previously unexpressed self-image of inferiority emerge, become less menacing, and no longer can repress the desire for a more balanced view of self) and social relationships (e.g., the patient's children release their own ambivalence and thereafter become more supportive). Those transformed cognitions, which themselves result from and in turn amplify altered feelings, contribute to a more adaptive, or more optimistic, or simply less self-defeating self. The restructuring of social relationships, a key feature of healing rituals in non-Western societies and sometimes an intended, sometimes an unintended part of psychotherapy, intensifies this process (cf. Turner 1967). As a result, catharsis transforms inner troubles as well as one's perception and experience of the local social world. A threatened and demoralized Taiwanese patient, for example, who fundamentally questions his sense of self-efficacy, accepts a shaman's master myth of a calm, reassuring, effective spirit commanding his consciousness. During the ritual treatment he enters trance and is possessed by the guiding spirit, during which time he expresses his fears in a crescendo of cathartic release authorized in the ritual setting. That emotional outpouring overwhelms lifetime repressions that were barriers to self-insight and in so doing renders this heretofore indocile man receptive to change at the core of his character. The patient comes to demonstrate in daily life the qualities of the mythic model: i.e., his self-image becomes that of the possessing deity, Buddhalike; he no longer sees the world as threatening and frustrating and beyond his ability to control. Through this powerful therapeutic experience, the patient reverses his negative cognitions, lessens anxiety and depression, and begins to transform his personality. As a member of the healing cult, moreover, his status is elevated and practical difficulties in his social life (e.g., too few clients for his woodworking business, and the absence of close friends to whom he can explain his fears of business failure and from whom he can receive affective support and practical advice) are overcome through his new social network (Kleinman 1980, pp. 333–352).

But catharsis and restructured social relationships are not the only therapeutic processes at work in this Taiwanese example or involved in symbolic healing generally. A deeply demoralized middle-class North American housewife accepts a cognitive behavioral model of her problem as a matter of the personally destructive effects of ideas of self-inefficacy which can be changed through a relationship with a therapist who applies an authorized protocol of behavioral interventions. The positive cognitions, like those of her Taiwanese counterpart, only here sanctioned by behaviorism's epistemology and experienced through the mediating symbolic meanings of the cognitive therapy, alter the patient's self-image and that activates the psychobiology of optimism and belief—i.e., change in neuroendocrine and autonomic nervous system activity experienced as decreased dysphoria, improved sleep and energy, and diminution in pain, weakness, and other symptoms (Hahn and Kleinman 1984; Tiger 1979). This is a model of social persuasion and learning; they too are at work in symbolic healing.

In the anthropological vision, the therapeutic relationship as a social exchange is important for such cognitive, affective, and physiological change to occur, which change may indeed be replicated in the patient's family setting and other intimate relationships (cf. Lewis 1971; Janzen 1978). In this model the contribution of improvement in relationships to therapeutic change is a concomitant or consequence of a more fundamental transformation in the meanings of those relationships that alters perception, expectation, communication, and commitment. Altered states of consciousness such as trance and other forms of dissociation—so ubiquitous outside the secular West—and transference, too, may facilitate these transformations. In the case of transference, the interpreted meanings are projected onto the healer, who comes to embody them; with altered states of consciousness, those resonant meanings are experienced by the patient in an aroused or highly focused ritual state which intensifies their effects and sanctions the transformation of self and social relationships.

Yet, in the cultural model of healing, these psychosomatic processes of change are not what is most essential about how symbols heal. The question is not whether catharsis or expectant faith or persuasion or restructured social relations is the single basis of healing. All are important, along with yet other processes of change—e.g., irony, paradox, modeling, insight—though none is determinative. It seems to be rather the dialectical structure of healing systems that is invariant. That structure creates a process of transformations that moves from cultural meanings to embodied experience, from the meanings of personal relationships to the relationships of personal meanings.

Psychotherapists who study healing are preoccupied with the content of particular kinds of healing systems and with proving that a particular mechanism of change (i.e., personal qualities of therapist, client expectations, or social learning) is universal. They are so absorbed by the mechanics of change (e.g., catharsis, confession, conditioning) that they fail to see that it is the structural organization of healing on the level of symbolic meanings that unifies all healing systems, psychotherapy included. The various mechanisms of psychophysiological and social change work within this universal symbolic structure, which, from the anthropological standpoint, is the source of cultural transformations of the body/self. Perhaps another way to put this difference in points of view is to say that psychotherapists have emphasized processes, while anthropologists have emphasized the systems within which those processes are lodged.

In summary, then, what is necessary for healing to occur is that both parties to the therapeutic transaction are committed to the shared symbolic order. What is important is that the patient has the opportunity to tell his story, experiences the therapist's witnessing of that account, believes the therapist's interpretation of his problems, and comes to use the same symbolic vehicles of interpretation to make sense of his situation. Because of his own need to believe and the rhetorical skills of the therapist to make key symbols relevant to the experience of the sufferer, the sick person becomes convinced that a transformation of his experience is possible and is in fact happening. On the level of psychotherapy as symbolic performance, as Tambiah has shown (1985), positive therapeutic outcome is enunciated and supported by the completion of the ritual transformation. The ritual ends, termination is justified, the myth is reenacted, symbolic harmony is achieved, the specific techniques and theories reach a logical and necessary conclusion, and therapist and patient agree that transformation has occurred. Even if there were no specific effect on pathology, patient and healer will feel better and believe in the efficacy of the treatment. That is to say, the therapist convinces the patient he has changed for the better and perhaps to do so needs to convince himself as well. But of course such powerful psychosomatic processes do alter pathology, even serious pathology.

To analyze the structure of healing is not to invalidate the experience or to accuse the healer of false consciousness. Quite the contrary. In this anthropological schema, healing is only possible because the relationship authentically particularizes personal experience in symbols that are culturally and practically relevant. That psychotherapy, like all indigenous systems of symbolic healing, is nonspecific neither diminishes its therapeutic significance nor invalidates its appropriateness for health care.

It is appropriate to inquire if the analysis of symbolic healing holds any practical implications for the training of the psychiatrist and other psychotherapists. Psychotherapy training tends to occur in the privacy of the psychiatric resident's experiences with his clients and clinical supervisors. The latter provide the therapist with a theory to interpret the patient's story and to plan his own actions. The supervisor introduces the novice psychotherapist to a particular "school" of psychotherapy. Since most psychotherapy supervisors are still psychoanalytically oriented, a psychoanalytic paradigm is what the resident learns. In principle, exposure to supervisors representing distinctive schools and participation in a seminar whose readings cover the different therapies should provide the resident with an overview from which he can later choose those theories and interventions with which he feels most comfortable and those methods with which his personal style is most consonant. In practice, most residents learn little about even the major alternative schools of therapy, and almost nothing about what is shared in the structural process of symbolic healing. Since psychotherapy is a lonely craft with uncertain standards, it is not surprising that young therapists feel a strong urge to affiliate with one of the schools (or, we might say, sects) in order to have colleagues who accept the same standards of "good" care.

I would suggest that a more systematic and useful means of teaching psychotherapy—to residents and also to graduate students in psychology and social work—is to begin with a seminar on symbolic healing cross-culturally that reviews what is known about universal and culture-specific aspects of symbolic healing and that explores the structural model of healing described above. This should provide the resident or the student with a broader, more critical understanding of the healing process. Following this, the major schools of psychotherapy can be compared and contrasted, with the explicit purpose of understanding those skills that are shared across schools and in the expectation that the trainee will develop familiarity with at least a few of the major therapies. Practical experience in patient care could mirror the didactic training. The resident would be supervised at first with the chief aim of helping him master the major therapeutic skills common to all systems of symbolic healing. Then the resident could be supervised in the different major therapies. Residents also need to know when one psychotherapeutic method may be more suitable than others for particular patients, because of the nature of their illness or their personality organization or their educational level and cultural background. If they do not practice the appropriate type of therapy for a particular patient, they should nonetheless be skilled in making suitable referral. The overall goal would be to organize a critical rational approach to psychotherapy (cf. Manschreck and Kleinman, eds., 1978; Manschreck and Kleinman 1981) that trains residents systematically in the most important skills (the building of rapport and trust, empathic listening, persuasion, remoralization, interpretation, etc.), that also educates residents to be critical readers of the psychotherapy literature on each of the major schools, and that offers each resident a framework for making sense of the major symbolic tasks of healing and for maximizing the symbolic effects of psychiatric care.

One desirable outcome of such a paradigm of training would be to force the profession of psychiatry to develop a more strenuous and systematic approach to psychotherapy, one that would be as independent as possible of the different therapeutic ideologies. At present, there is a tradition of important research on psychotherapy outcome, but there is no major comparative scientific study of the psychotherapies, nor for that matter any systematic empirical study of the use of a wide range of symbolic therapies by psychiatrists and other physicians. This is yet another paradox. Psychiatry is the home of psychotherapy in medicine, but, aside from promoting the important work of demonstrating that psychotherapy is useful, it has not taken this responsibility seriously enough to create a general scientific approach to psychotherapy and symbolic healing in medicine.

My analysis of psychotherapy points to a central tension in the relationship of the psychiatrist's care to medicine and health care generally that is the reciprocal of the challenge the psychiatrist's interest in the biography of the person and the social context of illness experience presents to medicine's dominant paradigm of clinical diagnosis and pathology.

The Paradox at the Heart of Health Care and Medicine

The *Shorter Oxford English Dictionary* defines paradox as "a statement or tenet contrary to received opinion or belief. . . . A statement seemingly self-contradictory or absurd, though possibly well-founded or essentially true" (p. 1428). Psychotherapy, the major form of symbolic healing in contemporary health care and biomedicine, illumines a postmodern paradox. Healing has become increasingly marginal to the West's dominant healing system.

The psychiatrist's psychotherapy is an anomaly in the house of scientific medicine, as is the family physician's and general internist's supportive, psychosocial care. Since the time in the Enlightenment when Bichat introduced the clinicopathological conference, with its central methodology of dissection of the cadaver of the dead patient, to determine the biological pathology as "the real cause" of the patient's problem and the focus of treatment, biomedicine has given research on disease a higher priority than the care of illness (Sullivan 1986). Biomedicine, and the professional health care sector of which it is the dominant component, is organized around specific biological investigations and treatment techniques that depend on increasing reductionism. Often such reductionism has been brilliantly successful, as in the treatment and prevention of infectious disease, or in the current revolution in our understanding of the molecular genetics of many heretofore mysterious disorders, e.g., Alzheimer's disease. But too often it has also encouraged medical approaches to the care of patients that have been inhumane and also ineffective (Eisenberg and Kleinman, eds., 1981). Talk therapy and the nonspecific (placebo) use of symbols are disdained. The psychiatrist, to the extent he is not thinking in neuroscience terms or employing somatic therapies, is an anachronism because he trades in general symbols, subjective meanings, and lived experiences.

Most of psychiatric care is not about the determination of brain pathology or the choice of a particular drug to cure the patient's disease, though these activities are not unimportant. The psychiatrist's work is chiefly about people's life stories. It is about aspirations and defeats, about passions and tragedies; in other words, it has to do with the deeply personal and life world (family, work, and school) problems that constitute the neuroses. And it is about assistance with the felt experience of illness in the gravest psychiatric disorders. Indeed, I would argue that this is psychiatry's signal contribution to medicine and health care generally: it has authorized the inner experience of the patient, the meanings of his illness, and his context of personal relationships as legitimate fields of inquiry and intervention for medical care.

Yet, under the pressure of culture change, psychiatry too is undergoing transformation (Eisenberg 1986). Academic psychiatry aims to become a version of high-technology internal medicine. Although the practice of psychotherapy continues to thrive in the clinic and private office because of the demands of consumers, the psychiatrist's concern with suffering and symbolic transformations is not well represented in medical schools or teaching hospitals.

The point is often made that psychiatrists, family physicians, and primary care internists should leave psychosocial inquiry and psychotherapy to other categories of health professionals—nurses, psychologists, social workers, physician assistants. This denigration of interventions that are not biological techniques (drugs, blood tests, endoscopes, surgical procedures) is reflected in the economic statuses of the psychiatrist and primary care practitioner, which are at the lowest end of the medical income scale, and in the limited curriculum time and research support provided for psychiatric teaching about symbolic interventions. One would think that every medical student should be trained to elicit the highest rates of placebo effects through mastery of nonspecific symbolic techniques. Far from it. Medical students are taught little else than that placebos confound clinical trials and may be unethical to provide without the consent of the patient. Hence the paradox. Biomedicine is the major system of healing in the West. Yet it has little to do with what is most central to most healing systems, symbolic healing. Indeed, it may not be an exaggeration to suggest that biomedicine is one of the only healing systems in which the structure of symbolic healing becomes most hedged in and routinely undercut and the training of the practitioner constrains her therapeutic use of meanings.

Whatever the doctor thinks she is doing (being scientific or providing the most up-to-date technology), she is nonetheless involved in a powerful set of psychological transactions with her patients. Her only choice is whether to recognize and maximize her "psychotherapy" or to be inattentive to it. To choose the latter is to fool herself (and her patients), and to lose some of her power to direct these psychological transactions toward conscious ends.

In this golden age of biomedical research and treatments, we are witnessing the problem of what shall become of symbolic healing. Perhaps, over the next century in North America, it will wither away in the profession of medicine, to be practiced only in the folk and popular arenas of health care. Perhaps it will continue to hang on as a marginal but inalienable aspect of psychiatry and the primary care professions, which themselves will be transformed into the high-technology image of the rest of medicine. This question must be asked of psychiatry per se: Can it continue to legitimate psychosocial problems, humanistic interests, symbolic interventions as medical concerns? If not, will psychiatry as we know it survive? Alternatively, is there the possibility that by opening these medical concerns to the human sciences (psychology, sociology, anthropology, history, philosophy, literary studies) —by doing these things that run against the grain, so to speak—that psychiatrists can make the meanings of illness experience and the social sources of human misery and symbolic healing an integral part of a more broadly conceived science of medicine and health care? I turn to this query as the penultimate of our anthropological questions for rethinking psychiatry.

Chapter 7

What Relationship Should
Psychiatry Have
to Social Science?

———————————◆———————————

. . . zoology, anthropology and psychiatry are really all one and . . . it is
perfectly natural to glide gently from one to the other via an interest in
patterns.

Gregory Bateson,
in B. Schaffner, ed.,
Group Processes

In recent years a biopsychosocial approach to medicine has captured public
interest and, within the medical profession, the attention of primary care
practitioners and psychiatrists. Yet most physicians still view biology as the
basic science of medicine. After all, medicine is glossed "biomedicine." I
think this is true of practicing psychiatrists too. We struggle to work out
models for relating psychological processes or the social environment to
disease, but ultimately we expect the answers to come from biology.

It comes as a surprise to many that social science, in fact, has had a long
relationship to medicine. A disproportionate number of the late-nineteenth
and early-twentieth-century founders of anthropology, sociology, and psychology were physicians. For example, W. H. R. Rivers, Paul Broca, and
Rudolph Virchow contributed significantly to the development of anthropology. Leading psychiatrists in this century—e.g., Emil Kraepelin, Sigmund Freud, Adolph Meyer, Aubrey Lewis, Karl Jaspers, Harry Stack
Sullivan—have had an interest in both cross-cultural research and anthropology. Major figures in modern anthropology—most notably, Alfred
Kroeber and Edward Sapir in the U.S., Bronislaw Malinowski and Meyer
Fortes in England, and Lucien Lévy-Bruhl and Claude Lévi-Strauss in
France—were in touch with developments in psychiatry, particularly psy-

choanalysis. Indeed, some, like George Devereux, were analysts. In the 1940s and 1950s, the "Culture and Personality" school of North American cultural anthropology brought together anthropologists and psychoanalysts in collaborative research. The development of social epidemiology of mental illness by Alexander Leighton, Morris Opler, and others was an outcome of these interdisciplinary ties, as were ethnographic studies of the psychiatric hospital as a small community by Jules Henry, William Caudill, Erving Goffman, and others. There is even a small cadre of psychiatrists, like myself, who are trained in anthropology and other social sciences, and a reciprocal group of anthropologists and social scientists of other stripes who work in psychiatry departments. Behavioral medicine has made the presence of psychologists more forcefully felt in medical schools, and departments of social and community medicine almost always employ sociologists. Yet for all their interaction, the reciprocal influence is quite limited, and social science in medicine is almost always regarded as a "new direction." The implication is that, unlike biological science, social science is marginal to medicine. When I was a first-year medical student at Stanford Medical School in 1962, social science teaching and teachers were greeted with stony ambivalence. That same response from beginning students greets social science teaching and teachers at the Harvard Medical School in 1987, a quarter of a century later, where I am myself a teacher of medical social science (Kleinman 1986, p. 223).

One might wonder if the social sciences contain knowledge and pursue questions which are irrelevant to illness and care.[1] This concern, fortunately, can be waved away almost immediately with a display of publications that disclose the salience of social forces in health and sickness and in medicine generally (Eisenberg and Kleinman, eds., 1981; Mishler et al. 1981; Fox 1980; Aiken and Mechanic, eds., 1986; Mechanic, ed., 1983, 1986). A very substantial amount of social science has been absorbed into medical research, where it forms the often unrecognized basis of biometry, epidemiology, health services research, psychosomatics, and social medicine. The language for formulating and assessing health policy, moreover, is increasingly that of economics and political science.

Why then, we might ask, do the social sciences remain marginal in psychiatry (and the rest of medicine)? There is, of course, the societal bias against social science, which spills over into the health professions. The crude articulation of this bias is the threadbare notion that social science is not a science, at least not in the same way biology is a science. Social science, in the rhetoric of Anglo-American political conservatives, is equated with the bête noire, socialism. The medical profession is not unaffected by this bias. There is also the bias of the entrenched biomedical model, which offers a stratigraphic view of disorder in which biology is the foundation, and psychological and social dimensions of sickness are seen as epiphenomenal, suprastructural layers to be stripped away to get at the infrastructural, i.e., biological, base. If a problem or intervention is specified in biological terms, it is scientifically legitimate. If it is described in the language of social science, it is scientifically suspect. Reductionism, viewed as an inadequate method in ecological and evolutionary biology, as I have already pointed out, flourishes in medicine. The everyday epistemology of medical sciences is that classical logical positivism discredited among philosophers of science but regnant in the halls of medical schools.

Ironically, at a time when primary care, social medicine, and public health disciplines are progressively introducing materials from social science into medicine, psychiatry has undertaken a voyage in the opposite direction. Psychiatry has long been the most important bridge between medicine and the social sciences, but the last decade has witnessed a romance with biology in psychiatry. Psychiatry has increasingly become inhospitable to social scientists.

But perhaps overt hostility in academic departments matters less than the attitudes of practitioners, which may be more receptive to social science. For after all, the same academic departments are inhospitable to psychoanalysis, which nonetheless manages to continue to flourish among practitioners in the form of more useful short-term psychodynamic psychotherapies. If the practical clinical relevance of social science were clearer, the interest of practitioners could be expected to grow, because the practicing psychiatrist knows he needs all the help he can muster, regardless of the source.

Requirements for admission to medical schools push students away from courses in the social sciences and give them inadequate preparation to absorb the relevant medical social science concepts and findings. Once in medical school, it is biological science, not social science, the student is expected to take seriously. The situation worsens after graduation. The expectation is that what is useful in social science can be acquired intuitively by the "sensitive" physician. Ill prepared to read the social science literature, the practitioner commonly is functionally illiterate when it comes to the basic terms, concepts, and modes of inquiry of the social sciences. Health science students also have few role models of clinicians who have expertise in the social sciences, whereas there are models galore of physicians who are basic biological researchers. As a result, the vast majority of medical students who will enter clinical practice receive no indication that social science is relevant to the day-to-day practice of clinical care. If this situation prevailed for biological science, it would quite properly be regarded as scandalous.

Unlike biological scientists, social scientists who are medical school faculty members can usually be counted on the fingers of both hands. They control a very small proportion of the teaching hours in the medical school curriculum and are generally allocated many fewer resources. This situation prevails in spite of evidence of the practical importance of social and behavioral science in the care of the large proportion of patients with chronic disorders and for the practitioner's understanding of major economic, political, institutional, and ethical constraints that are transforming medical practice (Starr 1983). Even though the lion's share of patient problems and of the daily concerns of most practitioners is consumed by these "soft" issues, they are devalued in the professional ideology when compared to those "hard" issues (biological research and interventions) that medical students, whatever their values upon entering the profession, soon learn to embrace as the pinnacle of biomedicine (Sullivan 1986).

I maintain that, with the exception of psychology, there has been no major influence of social science concepts on the clinical practice of psychiatry. Astonishing as it is to say, even highly pertinent psychological theory and research findings are neither taught to nor, in my experience, understood by psychiatrists (Kleinman 1986, p. 224).

Perhaps a final factor should be mentioned. Anthropology, as an example of critical theory in social science, has been called by one of its greatest practitioners, Sir Raymond Firth, the "uncomfortable science." Firth's idea is that anthropological analysis should lead the investigator (and his readers) to challenge common-sense understandings, unearth value conflicts and other hidden aspects of social life, assess the large-scale, changing historical and sociopolitical contexts of behavior, and self-reflectively confront the distortions in his own framework of analysis. The anthropologist, then, is always suspect, since he does not accept the psychiatry profession's paradigm as the only authentic account and turns the light of inquiry onto the practitioners themselves. For the anthropologist, furthermore, the patient's perspective is as salient as the professional point of view. Physicians feel uncomfrotable when social scientists reconfigure disease as social pathology or call the core value hierarchy of the profession to account by emphasizing the group over the individual, questions of social policy over those of the practitioner-patient relationship, health over disorder, and popular culture over medical culture. I list this problem because I wish to indicate the opposition it creates. In fact, I believe strongly that this line of questioning is appropriate and makes a positive contribution.

I think social science is marginal to biomedicine in large measure because of their very different paradigms of practice. For social science to develop a significant place in medicine will necessitate a transformation of the paradigm of practice, primarily of medicine, to a certain degree of social science too. We can see the beginnings of such transformation in schools of nursing and public health, but it has not yet begun in schools of medicine. Behavioral medicine should in principle be leading the way for social science in the clinic. In fact, it has established itself largely as a technologically oriented practice that complements biotechnology. Behavior, in its narrowest sense, is now a legitimate subject, alongside biology, in medical research and teaching; personal experience, social relationships, and cultural meanings—and the sciences that study them—are not yet fully legitimate (Kleinman 1986, p. 227).

Within the social sciences themselves there are additional barriers to an effective relationship with medicine. Most social scientists studying health problems have not acquired specific training in how to teach or research their subject, though a few postdoctoral programs now exist to offer such advanced education. There is still no systematic review of the social science literature, similar to that for biology, that identifies relevant concepts and methods and translates them into terms practically applicable in medicine. Funding for the social sciences in medicine exists only in the form of highly focused research grants that attempt to answer applied questions posed by physicians. Social science consultation is usually an effort to provide even more narrowly delimited assistance with statistical, research design, and instrument development questions. This neither attracts the very best social scientists to the health field nor allows those who are attracted to undertake long-term projects that can develop major conceptual models.

Moreover, just as physicians hold negative views of social scientists, social scientists possess stereotypes of health professionals that tend to be negative. A reverse ethnocentrism and romantic relativism in medical anthropology, for example, encourage a thoroughly tendentious view of folk healers as heterogeneous and beneficent and of biomedical practitioners as homogeneous and maleficent. For some medical sociologists of the antipsychiatry persuasion, psychiatrists are little better than jailers and the psychiatric profession an all-powerful leviathan. Medicalization is always evil. Teaching psychosocial skills to physicians can be excoriated as toadying to the power structure. Such ideological caricatures are clearly unhelpful. Marginal status, prejudice from the medical profession, and the lack of adequate resources and an appreciative audience are a few of the sources of this harmful bias. Happily, one sees less and less of it these days. Most medical social science is conducted at a fairly high level of professional competence by serious scholars who increasingly are making a long-term commitment to the health field and who have learned to relate to medical institutions without relinquishing the autonomy of a social science gaze.

A Model for the Relationship of Social Science and Medicine

Although the social sciences by and large have not had a great impact on medicine, their potential is great indeed, as I have tried to illustrate with the particular example of the relationship between anthropology and psychiatry.[2] In the early twentieth century, physicians were encouraged to go to the then new centers of excellence in biological science in order to obtain substantial training in research and teaching methods that they could bring back to enrich medicine. This group of academics became the critical cadre which transformed medicine into the modern engine of biomedical science. This could well be a model for the social sciences. That is to say, an appropriate model would view medicine as a profession based upon three sources of knowledge—biological science, clinical science, and social science. To remedy the frail status of the last of these sources of professional knowledge, various efforts would be undertaken to build a substantial relationship with social science. One of these steps would be the establishment of a few centers of excellence where major social science research and educational projects in the health field would be developed. Another would be the initiation of systematic monitoring of the social science literature for concepts and methods that might be useful to translate into practical professional models, research measures, and clinical techniques. A third step would involve the introduction of a sophisticated review of relevant social science theories and findings into the education of the general physician. Besides addressing clinical issues, introduction to social sciences would aim to educate the practitioner as a critical auditor of and contributor to the discourse on health policy, which is formulated in a language more akin to social science than to biomedicine.

To illustrate these possibilities, allow me to narrow this wide arena to the smaller stage I know best, the relationship of anthropology to psychiatry. I have argued that much is to be gained from a robust two-way relationship. Since I have used cross-cultural research as a case study, it might be held against me that I have taken precisely that subject where it is easiest to prove the case. What about the more difficult question of how anthropology can contribute to the training of the psychiatrist and to the clinical practice of the journeyman practitioner? Why should the busy psychiatry resident, who can barely keep afloat in a sea of practical details from his readings in the core of psychiatry and his immersion in clinical experiences, or for that matter the working psychiatrist, who daily struggles to hammer out improvised strategies that can integrate the humanity of patients' life stories with a scientific understanding of their disease processes—why should either pay serious attention to anthropology? What makes a serviceable anthropology for the clinician?

My answers come from my experience of teaching anthropology to psychiatry residents and fellows (and junior faculty) in several distinctive contexts: basic science seminars on psychiatric anthropology, lectures on anthropological aspects of pathology and treatment, and supervised clinical work in consultation-liaison psychiatry, cross-ethnic and cross-cultural community settings, and psychotherapy. These are not the only ways that anthropology can be taught; they are merely the practical, pedagogical methods that I have found most appropriate and effective. But first I will address a more basic question, what type of contribution should anthropology make?

There is no single answer to this question. Rather, an appropriate answer depends on the specific goals and contexts of particular psychiatric training programs and the needs of the practitioner. Based on these determinants, psychiatric educators and the self-directed clinician interested in learning what anthropology has to offer can pick and choose between several distinctive types of anthropological contribution.

Making Use of the Anthropological Data Base

Ethnographies can provide psychiatrists with detailed information about the social and cultural context within which their patients live and they themselves practice. Ethnographies provide basic descriptive data on social organization, including kinship and family systems, work and school settings, politicoeconomic practices, local community structures. In recent decades, ethnographies have often canvassed concepts of the person, coping styles, and ideas about and reactions to illness generally and mental illness in particular. Medical anthropologists have described local health care systems, especially their lay and folk sectors (e.g., Janzen 1978; Kleinman 1980; Lewis 1975; Lock 1980; Ohnuki-Tierney 1984). Psychological anthropologists have increasingly provided detailed findings on cognitive, affective, and behavioral processes (LeVine 1973; Levy 1973; Rosaldo 1980; Schieffelin 1976; White and Kirkpatrick, eds., 1985; Marsella et al. 1985). A recent surge of interest in what has come to be called psychiatric anthropology has extended the scope of such studies to include cultural beliefs about depression, bereavement, anxiety, and schizophrenia, and cultural influences on the ways emotions and mental disorders are experienced, including responses to psychiatric treatment (e.g., Estroff 1981; Scheper-Hughes 1979; Mullings 1984; Kleinman and Good, eds., 1985; Gaines 1979, 1982; Rhodes 1984; Low 1985; Guarnaccia et al. in press; Harkness 1987). For example, ethnographers have described the different idioms of distress that laymen use to express dysphoria—bodily complaints, images of natural phenomena like clouds and rain for depression, cosmological and kinship metaphors of distress. These idioms can confuse diagnosis, delay help seeking, and present problems in clinical communication and treatment if they are not understood (e.g., Nichter 1981; Parsons 1985; Rhodes 1984; Marsella and White, eds., 1982; Gaines and Farmer 1986).

Drawing on such studies, psychiatrists can begin to assemble for themselves an appreciation of how basic psychological and psychopathological processes are shaped by culture and social institutions. This information is central to diagnosis; it also can facilitate establishment of effective clinical communication and organization of appropriate therapeutic interventions. Where large numbers of the patients seen by psychiatrists come from different cultural groups or ethnic backgrounds, it is essential that psychiatrists master this background information (cf. Harwood, ed., 1981; Helman 1984). For many groups, it is feasible today to turn to the anthropological data base not only to understand distinctive child-rearing practices and core value orientations and behavioral rules, but even to obtain an overview of cultural influences on symptomatology, help seeking, treatment response, adherence, and other issues directly relevant to psychiatric practice. Yet for all its richness, it is discouraging to see how infrequently this data base is systematically drawn upon to provide psychiatric trainees and practicing psychiatrists with detailed knowledge of the context of distress and disorder. There are several lengthy bibliographies (e.g., Favazza and Oman 1977; Favazza and Faheem, eds., 1982; Kelso and Attneave 1981; Newton et al. 1982; Like ms.; Summerlin, ed. 1980), but these are not organized in a way that is easy for the busy clinician to utilize. The development of a streamlined computer program organized both by clinical topics and by ethnicity would be a major step forward that should be relatively easy to create based on the current state of medical anthropological knowledge.

The data base of anthropology and other social sciences also can be surveyed to address other topics relevant to the psychiatrist. For example, detailed information about social networks, mental health aspects of work and family life, and the structure of the local mental health system (formal and de facto) provide the psychiatrist with a better understanding of the social context of illness and care that can be developed for practical clinical assessment and for social policy and community health programs.

Applying Anthropological Methods in the Clinical Setting

Another contribution of anthropology to psychiatric practice is the use of its methods to elicit ethnopsychiatric beliefs of patients and families. The anthropological framework is useful to evaluate the influence of cultural rules on abnormal behavior. And anthropological methods can also improve cross-cultural and cross-ethnic communication in the clinical interaction (see Johnson and Kleinman 1984, in press). A variety of techniques can be used, several of which I will review later in this chapter. The point here is that techniques from ethnography can be applied in the clinic and the ward. These techniques can aid the psychiatrist in the interviewing process, his central clinical skill. Crucial to this skill is the work of interpretation. The psychiatrist must distinguish normal from abnormal, delusion from illusion, and determine the meaning of symptoms, their degree of severity, and their effect on the quality of life. As ethnography is at heart a hermeneutic endeavor, it should not surprise us that ethnographic skills can deepen and broaden the interpretive work of psychiatric doctoring.

Several examples described in Chapter 2 should illuminate the kind of contribution anthropology can make. Members of many American Indian groups believe, as we have seen, that shortly after the death of a loved one, the deceased's soul travels to the afterworld. On its lonely journey, the soul may turn toward the relatives it has left behind and call them to join it. Bereaved American Indians frequently experience the culturally normative illusion of hearing the soul of the deceased hauntingly call them. This is a deeply moving experience, but one that does not imply dire psychiatric consequences for the bereaved. Psychiatrists without knowledge of this culturally shaped expectation and the perceptual illusion it creates may mislabel the patient as delusional and prescribe antipsychotic drugs or hospitalize the individual, both of which will have negative effects. Traditionally oriented Hispanic Americans may dramatically display acute grief and other states of severe psychosocial stress with *ataques de nervios* (pseudoseizures and other dramatic bodily reactions) that are most often culturally prescribed normal behaviors, though they may at times represent pathology. Practitioners routinely overdiagnosis such behaviors as pathology (conversion disorder, the "Puerto Rican Syndrome") and prescribe treatments that are unnecessary, have toxicities, and interfere with normal coping processes.

Individuals from a wide range of cultures express psychological distress in a bodily idiom of distress that metaphorically conveys culturally appropriate meaning about their inner condition to those who understand the cultural idiom. Such somatization, as we have seen, is the norm worldwide, even in the more psychologically minded West. Neurasthenia in Chinese patients, *fatigué* afflicting French men and women, premenstrual complaints in North American women, and backache in North American men are common examples. But psychiatrists have frequently regarded this communicative system as "primitive," an "individual defense process," "pathological," and even a sign of a particular disease (e.g., depression, somatization disorder, or panic disorder). On the one hand, such a professional orientation encourages overdiagnosis and polypharmacy. Thus, chronic pain syndromes have been regarded as a "depressive equivalent," which means in practice that virtually all patients with this problem receive antidepressant medications, even though most will not benefit from these powerful therapeutic agents, which are not without significant side effects. On the other hand, a somatic idiom of distress (headaches, backache, constipation, dry mouth, fatigue) in major depressive disorder may impede the diagnosis of a treatable disorder, if the psychiatrist fails to appreciate those local cultural idioms of complaint that express emotional distress (for example, pressure on chest and into head *(men)* among Chinese, sternal discomfort among Portuguese Azorean immigrants, gastrointestinal complaints among Southeast Asian refugees in the United States, "heart distress" among Iranians).

Cultural and ethnic differences also routinely interfere with the diagnosis of other psychiatric conditions (generalized anxiety and other anxiety disorders, especially) as well as with compliance with the treatment regimen and other aspects of psychiatric care (Johnson and Kleinman 1984, in press; Katon and Kleinman 1981). Working with interpreters and with ethnic communities routinely creates or intensifies practical difficulties (miscommunication, serious faux pas in etiquette, and value conflicts) that can be better appreciated and dealt with through the use of anthropological methods (see Kaufert and Koolage 1984 and Harwood, ed., 1981). For a practial example, when working with interpreters, the clinician should first discuss in detail with the intepreter the questions she will use to evaluate the patient's mental status and the kinds of problems she is looking for. She should face the patient and family members, not the interpreter. The interpreter should be requested to describe the concrete content of the patient's speech in full, not simply to offer her own glosses. It is particularly important that the translator understand the psychiatrist is interested in and will not be judgmental about patient expressions of traditional beliefs, values, and behaviors which may strike the translator, precisely because they are traditional, as embarrassing or inappropriate, but which for the clinician are essential to distinguish the culturally normative from personal pathology. These strategies respond to expectable problems in working with translators that, when poorly handled, often lead physicians to either underestimate the effect of culture or to overestimate it.

The Place of Anthropological Concepts and Perspective in Psychiatric Education and Practice

Clinicians routinely use anthropological and other social science concepts without realizing it. "Culture," "social reality," "ethnicity," "social support," "social network," "labeling," "communication," "negotiation," to name an odd lot of examples, are more than merely common-sense terms; each is a concept tied to a research literature and has a history of technical usage in social science. Though they are part of the clinician's conventional wisdom, these terms benefit from interpretation. By more precisely defining these categories, the clinician can learn a more rigorous and systematic framework for analyzing psychosocial problems. He also begins to reflect self-critically on the process by which his professional culture and his own cultural background influence his thinking about distress and disorder. For example, stress is a Western folk model that has been "scientified" (Jacobson 1987). Much of the tacit knowledge about stress is folk wisdom that subtly biases the clinician (Young 1980). But there is an important technical literature on how stress, and social support, can be more effectively conceptualized and validly evaluated in individual lives and in family experience to provide practical aid to the practitioner (see, for example, N. Lin 1979, 1986; Kaplan, ed., 1983; Cleary 1987; Berkman 1981).

In the same way that biological terminology represents uncommon knowledge about the physical world, so too does social science terminology represent a heritage of uncommon knowledge about the social world. This body of knowledge can enrich the clinician's theoretical formulations as well as his practical judgment. This does not mean that all social science jargon is helpful; some simply rephrases, codifies, or, at worst, obfuscates common-sense knowledge. It is the understanding of key concepts and of the mode of reasoning that is important, not the memorization of social science terms.

Furthermore, awareness of the implicit, taken-for-granted conceptual orientations that influence our judgments about cases can lead us to reexamine our own categories and values (e.g., how we feel about gender differences, homosexuality, and other sexual practices, ethnic minorities, the disabled, the tortured). For this reason anthropological methods for eliciting others' points of view and comparing them with our own categories also hold the potential of teaching us how to become systematically aware of our own biases and prejudices—a role as therapeutically important to the general psychiatrist as it is to the psychoanalyst. A case in point is Dr. Kamin's failure to be self-critically aware of the influence of his personal and professional biases upon his evaluation of Dr. Smith in Chapter 5. Let me summarize what I take this anthropological sensibility and the methods that inculcate it in everyday practice to be about.

It is the cultural *pespective* itself, rather than any specific content, that is the most fundamental contribution anthropology can make to psychiatric education and practice. The essence of this perspective or vision can be summarized thus: The anthropologist seeks to understand the way his indigenous informants think about *their* world and *their* problems. He is respectful in the face of this alternative knowledge, treating it as comparable to, though different from, his own knowledge. Moving back and forth between lay and scientific perspectives, e.g., the self-understandings of his informants and his own interpretation of their experience, which may be quite different, the anthropologist's inquiry creates a dialectic between lived experience and its scientific observation. Out of this oscillation of meaning emerges a more valid, if always incomplete and augmentable, interpretation of how individual experience is culturally elaborated out of the stark existential crises that define our shared humanity.

When applied to psychiatric practice, this means that life story and illness experience should be integrated into the concern for disease process and the biology of behavior. And there should be a persistent movement toward reflective self-criticism of the cultural and institutional constraints limiting scientific judgment. This anthropological vision of the human condition, I hold, is of importance to psychiatry as a model of empathetic understanding of patients' predicaments. It can foster tolerance in valuing and responding to patient and family interpretations of these problems, as well as insight into the way local contextual processes contribute to illness. It can exemplify a more rigorous method for making clinical judgments and psychotherapeutic interpretations. Understanding the relation of meaning to behavior for the psychiatrist as much as for the anthropologist should involve a negotiation between lay and professional perspectives on the problem. It should also include a moral stance against oppression, degradation, and other forms of human misery. That which at first contact strikes the psychiatrist as culturally alien and repulsive must over time, if his care is to be responsive, be understood. Much will be accepted. That which cannot—i.e., the destructive, the illness-generating, the inhumane—must first be defined as such, and then interpreted for patients and families. After that, it is the mutual responsibility of the practitioner and the patient and family to deal directly with these aspects of culture, to try to change them or at the very least to ameliorate their effects. The contribution of anthropology to psychiatric education is not to instill a false romanticism toward all things cultural, but to insist that culture matters enough to become a central focus of analysis. Anthropology can liberate the psychiatrist from the blinders of too narrow a professional model of illness and care, and can encourage a perspective that is wider-angled, integrative, flexible, and sensitive to diversity, pluralism, and aspiration in the human experience. Anthropology, then, offers psychiatry a more critical but also more human image of the human condition.

A Program for Teaching Anthropology at Different Levels and in Different Contexts of Psychiatry

Introductory Level

Seminars covering the relevant anthropological literature should be introduced into the didactic course for first-year residents. Where a training program has a large ethnic patient population or where such a program is in a non-Western society, seminars should focus on key cultural values, behavioral norms and practices, styles of communication, and family and other social institutions that can significantly influence behavior. Information about the local social system, including its history and major problems, is an especially effective tool for providing students with an appropriate background for practice. Questions that review the normative life course—from child rearing to adolescence, from school to work careers, and from marital patterns to old age—may both enrich the psychiatrist's contacts with particular patients and be of practical clinical relevance to patient care (Clausen 1985).

Even in Western settings with limited ethnic populations, seminars can focus on studies of the core cultural orientation of the mainstream population and the local social ecology. The latter study must seek an understanding of the changing political and economic contexts of illness and practice, including formal and informal systems of social welfare, disability, health care, and other agents and agencies engaged in the negotiation of social problems. Besides the value of the specific content, trainees must be helped to become comfortable in reading anthropological materials and handling social science concepts and language. The introductory level is also where psychiatrists should learn how to critically read the mental health policy literature. Fostering attitudes that are sensitive to the importance of eliciting patient and family perspectives on the illness and treatment, and that are open to alternative points of view (religious, common-sense, etc.) is another objective.

Intermediate Level

For trainees in the middle of their psychiatric training, anthropology is most effectively taught in clinical settings, in the pragmatic context of patient care. For example, ethnic influence on the experience and expression of chronic pain is best learned while evaluating or treating ethnic patients with pain (Zborowski 1969; Lipton and Marbach 1986; Osterweis et al., eds., 1987). This knowledge is useful in assessing the degree to which cultural patterns of responding to pain influence symptom amplification (e.g., dramatic expression of distress, anxiety over latent meaning of symptoms, low threshold to pain) and acceptance of and response to particular treatments (such as psychotherapy, surgery, or acupuncture). Psychiatric ethnographies of the illness beliefs and behaviors of particular groups facing particular problems can be effectively read to answer these questions of ethnic influence.

Also of practical use are anthropological studies of patient and family values and expectations that create problems when the psychiatrist is insensitive to these aspects of clinical relationships and communication: for instance, when he breaks rules of etiquette, introducing linguistic and conceptual misunderstandings, failing to appreciate the extent to which the family is responsible for making decisions, among a long list of possible failings. Ethnic and cross-cultural patterns of help seeking and treatment by alternative healers also are best understood in the exigent, on-the-ground setting of caring for outpatients or inpatients. Alternative therapies may often be effective, but they also may delay more effective psychiatric treatment, produce noncompliance and dissatisfaction, and defeat comprehensive care. The pertinent anthropological knowledge can help the practitioner avoid such problems, which are often intensified, rather than lessened, by working through interpreters.

Clinical case rounds, clinical consultation with an anthropologist or cross-cultural psychiatrist, and special clinic or ward conferences on difficult diagnostic and management problems offer a more suitable forum to discuss the pertinent anthropological literature and its application to cases than didactic conferences (Smilkstein et al. 1981; Kleinman 1982). The latter may be useful, however, for a more methodical review of large cultural issues, such as somatization of mental disorders and other cultural idioms of distress, normal trance and possession states, culture-bound syndromes, cross-cultural influences on personality, and routine culturally based conflicts in clinical care that pose significant local problems.

One very effective pedagogic technique is to require psychiatric trainees to make supervised home visits to their patients' communities so that they can have the experience of participant-observation, if ever so briefly, in the local cultural context. After such visits, debriefing by an anthropologist can help in generalizing from concrete experience. Similarly, visits to the local disability system offices and to those of alternative practitioners or folk healers who are routinely consulted by patients can be a useful way not only to teach about the powerful influence (positive and negative) of the larger social welfare and health care systems, but also to help neophyte psychiatrists to come to terms with ingrained biases which reflect differences in class, ethnic, religious, and educational backgrounds. The result of such experiences is to give the resident a feeling for ethnography, so that in his case formulations he will aspire to include mini-ethnographies of the effect of the patient's life world on his experience of illness.

The creation of a mini-ethnography of the patient's experience of illness is based on an interpretation of the patient's and family's narrative of the illness. The clinician draws on systematic knowledge of the patient's life world and personal biography to interpret the significance of the story of the illness for the patient, the family and significant others, and for the clinician himself. The psychiatrist does this by analyzing the various accounts of the illness with respect to their major plot line, metaphors, and the rhetorical devices employed to tell the story of the illness from onset, through exacerbations and treatment contacts, up to the time of the most recent encounter. The mini-ethnography goes back and forth between story and local context to understand personal experience and its social sources and consequences. By recording the chief elements of the mini-ethnography either in the patient's official psychiatric record or in his own private notes, the clinician has the opportunity to revise, add to and rework his interpretation in light of new information. His purpose is to use the mini-ethnography as the background against which to make sense of later experiences and especially problems in care. The report of the mini-ethnography is the appropriate material from which supervisors can assess the trainee's practice and particularly his skill in clinical interpretation. (For a detailed description of such mini-ethnographies see Kleinman, 1988).

The trainee's clinical interviews should be supervised for evidence of skills in eliciting patient and family explanatory models of illness (Kleinman 1980). In such supervision, residents should also learn to describe and conceptualize culturally based problems affecting the patient and his family's perception of symptoms and communication of distress and coping responses. (Kleinman, Eisenberg, and Good 1978; Katon and Kleinman 1981; Johnson and Kleinman 1984). This is also the appropriate setting for residents to acquire competence in working through translators.

Patients' explanatory models of illness usually respond to such personal and family concerns as "Why me?" "Why now?" "What is wrong?" "How long will it last and how serious is it?" "What problems does it create for me?" "How do I get rid of this problem? That is, what will make me better?" Patients' and families' models of treatment often express concerns about the appropriateness, efficacy, and side-effects of medication and other therapies. Cultural models may implicate sacred or secular causes and treatments; they also tend to relate personal distress to social circumstances. Patients may believe that they are victims of sorcery or witchcraft, or have broken a taboo, or that for religious or other reasons they cannot accept medical advice and treatment (Weiss et al. 1986). Blumhagen (1982) showed that North American hypertensives often believe their disorder is too much tension, not high blood pressure, and thus they take their medicine only when they feel tense. Rhodes (1984) learned that medicine for chronic schizophrenic patients may not be taken because of the metaphors patients use to understand what medicines do: control the mind, turn off creativity, sap strength, provide "artificial" rather than "natural" support. Helman (1981) discovered that patients in his primary care practice in England view psychotropic medication as "food" or "fuel" which influenced their judgments about when to follow medical advice and when to challenge the practitioner. Nations and her colleagues (1985) found, in a primary care clinic serving a poor rural population in Virginia, that many patients held popular cultural views of their illnesses and treatments that differed substantially from those of their doctors. Such popular illness terms in this population—e.g., "sugar," "high blood," "nerves"—were usually not known by the medical staff, even though these explanatory models significantly shaped inappropriate help seeking, nonadherence to the medical regimen, clinical miscommunication, and patient and physician frustration with care. The elicitation of patient explanatory models should be a routine part of psychiatric care and can help obviate these problems.

Working through interpreters, for reasons I have previously noted, always carries with it the possibility of introducing serious distortion (see the second case illustration in the Epilogue). Asking interpreters to describe precisely patients' explanatory models, no matter how traditional or different (and therefore to many assimilated interpreters irrelevant or embarrassing) they sound, can aid in protecting against such distortion. To elicit explanatory models, the psychiatrist asks the patient what his view is of the etiology, reason for onset at a particular time, pathophysiology, course, and expected and desired treatment. She can then systematically compare patient (and family) models with her own to detect major sources of conflict. Negotiating with patient explanatory models can prevent tacit conflicts from interfering with patient care (Rosen and Kleinman 1984). The clinical setting is also the proper place to teach residents how to assess family and work problems, and social support, and how to help patients relate to relevant social agencies. The expectation should not be that this is the work of the psychologist or social worker, because these are core skills required for all mental health professionals. Indeed, they should be taught to medical students and primary care physicians, who provide much of the care in the de facto mental health system (Regier et al. 1978).

Rotation of residents through community mental health programs should have anthropological or other social science input. For these are opportunities to learn ethnographic skills and obtain local cultural insights crucial to the practice of psychiatry. This is the appropriate setting in which to foster negotiation skills with local agencies and informal community groups that enable psychiatrists to learn how to bridge the gap between the culture of patients and the professional culture of the mental health field. Here one learns that barriers to effective care arise as often from the latter culture as from the former; and one can also gain practical experience identifying and removing these cultural obstacles.

This community experience is the right background against which to teach trainees about social ecological sources of distress and preventive interventions. In order to teach in such settings, either anthropologists (or other social scientists) must possess clinical experience or they must teach conjointly with clinicians who have a social science background. In North America, there is now a cadre of psychiatric teachers with social science training who are able to more effectively bridge psychiatry's clinical and social science bases. My experience is that they are often more effective in conveying cultural influences on the shaping of illness and the response to treatment than they are in clarifying the social origins of alienation and demoralization in local contexts of power that differentially transmit the effects of macrosocial forces to individuals. This aspect of social epidemiology can be more effectively taught by immersion in local community contexts in which lack of support and inadequate resources magnify stresses. This is also the appropriate place to try out small-scale sociotherapies (e.g., support groups, urban survival skill workshops, educational programs in ethnic agencies, therapeutic programs in school or work place, home visits) and to pilot highly focused preventive interventions for at-risk populations (e.g., suicidal adolescents, family members of chronic patients, refugees with a history of adaptational problems and repeated traumas, the homeless). Each psychiatric trainee should be required to have experience either in personally developing or working with an existing local preventive intervention project.

Learning to do psychotherapy might follow the suggestions offered in the last chapter for creating a comparative framework to study the major forms of psychotherapy and to develop key therapeutic skills shared by all systems of symbolic healing. The former, I have already suggested, could be accomplished in the setting of a seminar that reviewed various approaches to psychotherapy in the framework of comparative analysis of healing systems cross-culturally. Clinical supervision could be oriented to the development of therapeutic skills determined to be universal in the healing process—i.e., development of personal warmth, genuineness, trust, and rapport and fostering of catharsis, empathic witnessing and social persuasion, problem solving, emotional support, remoralization, and interpretation. A systematic determination of core skills and education in their mastery would be a revolutionary change in the usually haphazard and often ideological way psychotherapy is currently taught. Evaluation of clinical competence could also be targeted to assess the acquisition of this battery of culturally informed attitudes and skills.

Advanced Level

Whereas all psychiatric trainees should have instruction at the beginning and intermediate levels only those with a special interest in cultural issues will want more advanced instruction. Here the possibilities are considerable. Reading courses can be set up with psychiatric or psychological anthropologists on topics of the trainees' choosing—e.g., child development cross-culturally; child abuse in particular cultural contexts; suicide, alcohol and drug abuse, adolescent problems, and so forth among ethnic groups; the cross-cultural data base on depression, anxiety disorders, or schizophrenia; cultural aspects of psychotherapy or psychopharmacology; comparative analysis of healing systems. Alternatively, interested trainees should be encouraged to take relevant courses in the anthropology departments of their institutions or of neighboring ones.

I favor reading courses that support trainees' efforts to do small (archival or field) research projects that can be critically evaluated and written up for publication as research papers. I think this is especially important in non-Western societies, where trainees' research can help make psychiatric diagnostic and treatment approaches culturally valid. Hence critiques of DSM-III and ICD-9 that point out the problems in their use with particular cultural and ethnic groups, as well as critiques of the psychometric instruments based on these nosologies, can aid local programs to develop more culturally appropriate disease taxonomies and diagnostic criteria.

Advanced training can take the form of postdoctoral fellowships and M.A. and even Ph.D. programs. But for most trainees with this interest, simply doing focused reading and conducting a literature review and small pilot study should be sufficient. One question deserves special attention:

since psychiatry's knowledge base and treatment systems are derived from Western culture, what changes need to be introduced to render psychiatry appropriate for local populations? That is, what is needed to create a Chinese, an Indian, an African, a Papua New Guinean psychiatry? Here focused ethnographies by advanced trainees of the local mental health system and of the local social system within which its patients dwell can complement critical reviews of the international literature in psychiatry to contribute to the building of such culturally appropriate psychiatry.

Special Situations

Cultural and anthropological training are especially valuable for professionals working with refugees and migrants, who are under heightened risk for illness and for culturally induced problems in health care. Courses, clinical supervision, and collaborative cross-cultural research projects can be devised to provide basic information on these high-risk groups useful for local preventive and therapeutic programs. These educational experiences can also help trainees assess their own cultural perceptions and experiences and their effects on their clinical practice (see Spiegel 1976; E. H. B. Lin 1984; K. M. Lin 1979). For trainees who are themselves recent immigrants from non-Western cultures undergoing the acculturation process, educational experiences that focus on problems of acculturation and cross-cultural communication can be an unrivaled means of confronting their own problems and mastering techniques useful for effective cross-cultural care.

Again, the purpose of training is to focus on the practical issues requiring anthropological assessment as a means of teaching about highly relevant cultural influences as much as for solving specific clinical problems. Anthropology should help trainees conceptualize problems in the cross-cultural care of particular patients and thereby generalize from those cases to this category of problems in patient care. There is a pertinent literature in medical anthropology that describes practical techniques to improve assessment of health problems among members of non-Western refugee and recent immigrant groups as well as respond to common barriers to effective cross-cultural communication generally. This material should be mastered by trainees who are routinely faced with cross-cultural and cross-ethnic questions. But engagement with anthropology's ideas about cultural relativism can help liberate all trainees from professional biases and the tendency to dehumanize inherent in socialization in bureaucratic rational-technical paradigms. Finally, those trainees with a special interest in international psychiatry should also learn to be informed users of anthropological concepts and findings, especially since anthropology is increasingly being called on to address the major international health problems.

Anthropology for the Practicing Psychiatrist

The practitioner daily confronts challenges to his sense of clinical competence. Psychiatric practice is a lonely experience with few clear-cut benchmarks of success or failure. If the professional becomes demoralized by perceiving inadequate mastery over professional knowledge and skills, the impact on his care of patients can be profound. This is an element in the complex of frustrations referred to as burn-out. But all neophyte practitioners of psychotherapy are at special risk for this problem, since they experience a gnawing recognition that no board examination, no academic degrees, and no set of therapeutic experiences can establish whether the care they give is of high quality. The problem is not so much in themselves, as it is in their profession's failure to come to terms with the need for a comparative standard of competence that crosses the narrow sectarian lines of particular schools of psychotherapy. I believe it is for this reason that many practitioners eventually choose to enter a sectarian school, even though they may at first have been as critical as others of the limits and dangers of a narrow orthodoxy. By entering a particular school, a psychiatrist circumvents the existential crisis of competence; he exchanges the wearying effect of uncertainty for the buoying belief there is one certain way of doing psychotherapy that can be affirmed by a circle of peers who share the same standards.

A comparative analysis of healing systems together with a practical framework for understanding and applying what are universal tasks of healing could be of singular value to the young psychiatrist. They could provide him with a critical method to assess the claims and approaches of new therapeutic movements, to routinely evaluate and reform his own practice, and to measure his career development in the mastery of a lifetime craft. In the same vein, a usable anthropological methodology to audit and interpret the patient's story of the illness would supply the psychiatrist with the sense that there is, side by side with the analysis of psychiatric disease, a disciplined approach to the assessment of illness experience and life history. And, indeed, such a clinical methodology is to be found in medical anthropology (cf. Kleinman, 1988).

For assessing illness meanings, anthropological theories of language, metaphor, and interpretation and especially an appreciation of ethnography can be very helpful (e.g., Geertz 1973, 1984; Sahlens 1976; Tambiah 1985; Moore 1978; Lakoff and Johnson 1980; Clifford and Marcus 1986; Rosaldo 1980; Turner and Bruner, eds., 1986). An anthropological model of illness, as an example, identifies four major types of illness meanings that should be assessed by the psychiatrist (Kleinman 1988). *First*, there are the conventional meanings of symptoms. Here metonymy or metaphor may create a double entendre expressing emotional distress through somatic complaints. Phrases that signal severity of symptoms, imagery used to communicate course and duration of complaint, and lexical terms (especially adjectives) that elaborate on the brute materiality of a complaint—all give the practitioner entrée into the patient's perception and experience of illness. Inasmuch as we learn conventional ways of complaining (e.g., about pain, weakness, dis-ease) as members of a social group, the assessment of symptom meanings needs to include an appreciation of a group's concepts of normal and abnormal behavior. Are the members of a social group relatively expressive or inhibited? What major communicative codes and rhetorical techniques do they employ? Which models of illness behavior (i.e., how to act when sick) are most salient? What patterns of help seeking prevail? And which are the complaints that carry special cultural significance?

The *second* type of illness meaning is the powerful (often stigmatizing) significance of culturally salient disorders—e.g., AIDs in present-day North America; major mental illness in China today and in the past; tuberculosis in nineteenth-century Europe; cancer in the twentieth century in Europe and North America; afflictions owing to witchcraft in Africa; soul loss syndromes in a variety of societies; and all the other culture-bound syndromes that preoccupy members of societies everywhere. These illnesses bring particular constellations of meanings to the sick person, meanings that menace and demoralize and may change forever the patient's life course. Think of how a diagnosis of leprosy in South Asia turns a sick person into a pariah, or how the label of mental retardation humiliates and spoils the self-identity of children and adults in North America who struggle throughout life to maintain a "cloak of competence." Knowledge of these meanings and how they are embodied in the patient's experience can come from key readings from the literature in medical anthropology and related social sciences (and from key works of fiction).

The *third* type of illness meaning is the significance that a chronic illness takes on in the life world of the patient. Here ethnographic appreciation of the way social context shapes experience is a crucial complement to psychodynamic formulations of the intrapsychic significance of a chronic disorder. Chronic illness is enacted in relationships, from which it draws significance and to which, recursively, it contributes meanings. Illness changes context; context alters illness. All too often the context is left out of psychiatric interpretations of illness experience. The best way for the psychiatrist to bring it in is to read how first-rate ethnographers (and for that matter biographers too) accomplish this, how they understand the person in webs of relationships, how they capture the essential features of setting and activities. There is a wealth of relevant social science information on the way work, family, and other social settings along with gender, age, and ethnic background influence illness behavior, information which can enrich psychiatric assessment and enhance treatment. The introduction of such material must not be used to overwhelm the practitioner, but merely to suggest new directions for the possible development of his clinical interest and for his own continuing intellectual growth.

Finally, there are the explicit explanatory models of patients, families, and practitioners to which I have referred in outlining an educational program for residents. Here the practitioner may choose to learn a new technical skill (i.e., elicitation and negotiation of explanatory models—Johnson and Kleinman, in press) in order to provide a more thorough psychosocial assessment.

This schema of illness meanings can be elaborated into a series of clinical strategies that the practitioner can apply (Kleinman, 1988), but the real value of such an anthropologically informed methodology is not the prescription of cookbook-style techniques, for after all the audience is experienced clinicians. Rather it is the style of the ethnographic approach itself which should be of value as a general guideline for how to explore this important, though usually tacit, clinical topic: the nature and implications of meanings within the experience of illness and the trajectory of care. That is to say, ethnography, as I have already shown, can become a model for that aspect of clinical practice having to do with the patient's, the family's, and even the practitioner's *experience*. Other anthropological concepts, methods, and data that I have reviewed as elements in the education of the trainee psychiatrist may also be pertinent to the continuing medical education of the practitioner. Certainly, practitioners may feel the need for other intellectual skills (e.g., terms and concepts from political science and economics) to more effectively audit and contribute to the discourse on mental health policy, locally and nationally.

Heretofore, practicing psychiatrists have not been attracted to international health in the same numbers as their colleagues in other medical specialties, but there is reason to suspect this interest will become more important to psychiatrists in the final decade of this century, as psychosocial aspects of tropical disease and the current international epidemic of violence due to substance abuse together with the burden of major mental illness in developing societies figure more prominently in international health priorities. Here again social science attitudes, knowledge, and skills are of substantial value (Weiss 1985).

There are, of course, very real limits to what social science can accomplish. An overly mechanical application of the anthropological method (or of that of sociology or social psychology) can be as dangerously dehumanizing as an overly narrow biomedical vision. Too much attention to the intended and unintended consequences of social process can paralyze the actor. The clinician, for all his need for insight, is expected to act, and to do so in exigent circumstances. The therapeutic mandate is not part of the social scientist's professional experience. Also, if not appropriately introduced to the relevant literature, the practitioner may feel lost and frustrated, as he turns from the writings of anthropologists to the quite different approaches of sociologists, political scientists, and economists. Social science inquiry in and of itself can disclose only a portion of the causal web that creates or exacerbates most disorders; to complete the picture, it is necessary to complement studies of the changing social sources of morbidity and chronicity with biomedical research. The same, of course, is true for treatment and prevention: analysis of the social basis of psychiatric care tells only part, albeit a very important part, of the story of healing. Finally, there are problems in psychiatry—e.g., diagnosis of organic brain disorders, or treatment of metabolic and endocrine disorders like diabetes and hyperthyroidism that cause acute episodes of depression or psychosis, or emergency management of life-threatening drug intoxication—that are neither elucidated by social science knowledge nor resolved by practices informed by that knowledge. But to my mind these are relatively minor cautions. In my experience, the benefits of a social science vision in clinical practice greatly outweigh its limis and costs. Indeed, this vision encourages a refreshing sense of humility, which is the obverse of the hubris that regrettably characterizes so many new clinical modalities and is widely recognized as the clinician's nemesis. When compared with biomedical iatrogenesis, which has become commonplace, iatrogenesis in psychiatry based on social science has not been a significant problem.

Not all of the educational experiences I have outlined may be appropriate for a particular practitioner. The purpose is not to make the practitioner into an anthropologist or sociologist, but rather to enrich practice and perhaps also the life of a practitioner with a perspective and practical skills informed by social science that can advance the application of highly pertinent interdisciplinary concepts in the hurly-burly of clinical work. Not the least of the benefits is the potential such a perspective holds to remoralize practitioners who must face the wearying demands of practice, especially those who practice in communities quite different from their own sociocultural background or in social settings that sharply constrain distribution of resources and that severely circumscribe the physician's work.

As for the potential of anthropology and other social sciences to contribute to the academic side of psychiatry, the first five chapters of this volume suggest numerous ways that a social science line of inquiry and program of research as well as anthropologists and other social scientists themselves can, and do, contribute. Research support for social scientists, especially anthropologists, working on psychiatric subjects and for psychiatrists employing ethnography and other social science methods has not been adequate.[3] In spite of this obstacle, if we use anthropology again as our example, we see that a number of anthropologists have pursued long-term research projects on the sources and forms of mental llness and psychiatric care. (An excellent example is Robert Edgerton's [1984] work over a quarter of a century to build a program of anthropological studies of the mentally retarded in society. Other examples include Vincent Crapanzano 1973; Atwood Gaines 1979; Sue Estroff 1981; Spero Manson, ed., 1982; Jane Murphy 1964, 1982; Byron Good 1977; Robert LeVine 1973; Robert Levy 1973; John Kennedy 1987; Nancy Scheper-Hughes 1979, 1987). There is more research today on ethnopsychiatric concepts and practices in different ethnic groups and cultures than ever before. Anthropological approaches are also enriching clinical, epidemiological, and evaluation studies. The chief weaknesses have been the limited elaboration of autonomous anthropological theories about the relationship of culture and psychiatric disorder and the lack of a wider audience within the profession. One aim of this volume is to advance such a theory and attract such an audience.

If I canvassed sociology or social psychology for other examples, the numbers of scholars working on mental illness and psychiatric care would, of course, be much greater (see, for example, relevant bibliographies in Mechanic, ed., 1983; Eisenberg and Kleinman, eds., 1981; Elliott and Eisdorfer 1982; Gove 1975; McHugh and Vallis, eds., 1986; Mishler et al. 1981). Sociologists and social psychologists have conducted studies on almost every aspect of mental health and illness, with scholars devoting entire careers to the study of subjects of direct importance to psychiatry, again under the substantial constraint of very limited funding. In spite of this fact, much of the most original and important research on the psychosocial sources of illness and chronicity, which I have cited in this book, has been produced by sociologists and social psychologists.

It must be reemphasized that the materials I have chosen to canvass represent my own involvement with anthropology and cross-cultural research, and are not meant to represent the rich variety of social science, or even all of anthropological work on illness and care. There is also the danger that this review, because I have tried to engage so many aspects of psychiatry, will be read as a program for a radical reform of all of psychiatric education and practice, an evangelical vision of a utopian future. That is definitely not my intent. While I do believe the key questions raised in these chapters should challenge the way we think of psychiatric categories, diagnosis, and the influence of the profession's values on the work of the practitioner, I do not believe anthropology or social science at large can specify a program of major reform, or that such reform would necessarily be desirable. What the seven questions I have asked in these chapters and the Epilogue that follows can do is to structure a critique of key aspects of psychiatry. They can be the source of a challenging perspective and data base that help professionals rethink certain of the great questions that make psychiatry such an exciting field of practical problems in the human sciences, problems that also frustrate psychiatry's practitioners and academicians. Although I have outlined a large number of ways that the relationship between psychiatry and social science, and more particularly anthropology, can be enriched, I anticipate that there will only be a few centers that will have the interest and manpower to develop a serious program. Even for these academic centers my objective is modest. After all, what I have argued for is theory building and empirical research and experiments in the education of psychiatrists, tasks which lie ahead, tasks whose outcome cannot yet clearly be predicted. But I also believe that various of the ideas I have discussed are well enough elaborated and supported by research that they can now become part of the professional discourse throughout psychiatry.

The reciprocal question deserves a brief comment. Why should social scientists be interested in encouraging this relationship? What conceivable contribution can psychiatry make to anthropology or the other social sciences? No substantial interdisciplinary relationship can sustain the flow of work solely in a single direction. Fortunately, there is a rather specific set of opportunities that psychiatry can offer social scientists. It is important to recognize that social science, again employing anthropology as our example, is in a peculiarly transitional phase in its own trajectory. The study of small-scale preliterate societies has moved from the center of the discipline of anthropology to its margins. The study of developing societies and of postindustrial nations has engaged anthropologists in applied areas of research—e.g., agriculture, health, social development per se, the problems of ethnic minorities and refugees. Indeed, developing nations, quite properly in my view, have increasingly required that in order for anthropological research by foreign investigators to be approved, it must make some sort of practical contribution to the understanding and resolution of local social problems. Studies of kinship, which dominated the field for 100 years, have given way to studies of migration, urbanization, specific community health problems, and the kinds of issues I have reviewed in this book. In each of these areas, conceptual issues come to the fore that expand anthropology's theoretical horizon. Thus, one reason psychiatry is of importance to anthropology is that it turns out to be a surprisingly good subject to rethink from a cultural standpoint and thereby to connect anthropological theory to a much wider set of conceptual concerns. For a discipline searching for a way out of traditional intellectual debates that have become something of a blind alley—e.g., the nature of so-called primitive society and thought, which has remained a question at the heart of the discipline for the past 100 years (Kuper 1987)—psychiatry is a boon. For a discipline searching for linkages to practical issues of large moment in the current world, psychiatry is filled with opportunities. Psychiatry also has the more mundane significance of opening up job opportunities and access to a wider range of funding sources. The cross-cultural materials that I have reviewed should also indicate that psychiatric themes are increasingly taking on importance in the international health arena. As non-Western societies rethink their priorities in inviting foreign anthropologists to conduct field work, practical benefits, such as those that can result from mental health studies, will increasingly determine which projects are approved and which rejected. The very rapid development of studies in the anthropology of health and illness as one of the more robust directions in anthropology and the resurgence of interest by international organizations in anthropological studies on the major tropical diseases offer further evidence that medicine and psychiatry are now important and are likely to develop even greater importance for anthropologists.

Were I to canvass sociology or social psychology, we would encounter many of the same issues. Mental health problems and psychiatric care and social welfare systems have become central concerns to these disciplines. Indeed, these subjects are more central to these other social science disciplines than they are to anthropology. Mental illness and psychiatry not only are relevant applied topics for research but hold significance for development of theory and research methodologies too (see relevant chapters in Fiske and Shweder, eds., 1986). Moreover, many more sociologists and social psychologists than anthropologists find employment in the health and mental health fields. Thus, these fields are of rather substantial significance to the social sciences.

I have asserted that social science should have a more robust, two-way relationship with psychiatry. I recognize, however, that this relationship could become even more marginal over the next decade in view of the retrenchment of the current period. If the relationship should weaken further, that will be to the detriment of both disciplines and to solving the major mental health problems of our times. In the event, what is important is that this relationship as much as the particular questions I have raised should be more broadly debated by psychiatrists and social scientists.

Epilogue

They said, "You have a blue guitar,
You do not play things as they are."

The man replied, "Things as they are
Are changed upon the blue guitar."

Wallace Stevens,
"The Man with the Blue Guitar"

There are three sets of images out of my experiences as a psychiatrist and as an anthropologist studying psychiatry that dramatize the need for and uses of a culturally informed psychiatry. These images also are graphic descriptions of the substantial barriers that continue to block the effective introduction of the approach described in the preceding chapters into the profession of psychiatry. The first image illustrates a seventh and final question about psychiatry, what role can psychiatry play in international health? Heretofore, psychiatry's contribution to the changing burden of health problems in developing societies has been minimal. Yet the prevalence in those societies of mental health problems is substantial and growing. Schizophrenia, depression, substance abuse and its violent consequences, the psychiatric conditions caused by parasitic disease and malnutrition, and the psychological sequelae of forced uprooting and ethnic conflict are only a few of the global health problems that point up the potential relevance of psychiatry and the other mental health professions for poor populations in the less economically and technologically developed societies.

167

I

The first picture is a common example of psychiatric practice in the Third World. The scene keeps shifting among psychiatric facilities I have visited in urban China, rural India, and Indonesia. Although this example comes from a particular rural clinic in India, the conditions are similar enough to those in many other developing societies: a simple clinic building, one large waiting area—poorly lighted and ventilated, with a few old wooden benches and a rickety desk or two—filled with a very large number of patients and their families in native dress. There are pungent, earthy smells. There is much noise. Here and there an acutely psychotic patient breaks into song or screams incoherently; everywhere family members are talking; over by one wall an elderly woman squats on the tamped dirt floor, her head in her hands, tears slowly coursing down her cheek; on the opposite side of the waiting area, an adolescent boy withdraws from the touch of his father and shakes his head negatively at a request from his sister. Two small rooms stand on either side of the waiting area. In each a psychiatrist sits at a desk speaking to a patient and his family members and friends. Each room is packed with people, including both patients waiting to be seen and those who have already been interviewed but for whom there is a prescription to be filled or a blood test to be taken. A single nurse and her two young assistants attempt to quiet the onlookers and to get some of them to leave.

The psychiatrist has begun an interview. First, he looks around the room, then at his watch; it is midway through a four-hour clinic session. He has already seen eight to ten patients, and as many remain to be seen, including a large agitated man who keeps walking in and out of the room glaring at the psychiatrist, brushing off the restraining hands of coworkers and nurse. The psychiatrist looks back at the patient sitting before him. He realizes he has missed her opening words. Now she launches into a story that he cannot follow. He starts asking questions. The patient's father begins to answer. "No let your daughter respond," he says irritably. The psychiatrist thinks, How can I possibly get through the rest of the cases? The patient begins again, telling a story of an embarrassing school failure. The psychiatrist is impatient. The story strikes him as superficial and irrelevant. He can't wait for her to describe the episode in its entirety, so he asks abruptly, "Well, what happened? Tell me directly, I can't take all day! Is this the real reason you came today?" The patient looks hurt and is silent for a moment. The psychiatrist sees that she is fighting to hold back tears. Her father prods her: "Go on, tell him the problem. He is a busy doctor, and he is not a fortuneteller who can guess what you are thinking." The patient looks at the floor, crestfallen. "That's all right," says the psychiatrist in a gentler voice. "I am waiting. I see that you are upset; tell me what it is."

All of a sudden with a rush of emotion a series of words of such intense suffering break out from the frail young woman that all eyes in the crowded room rest on her, all the whispered conversations stop. Now she begins a different, deeply personal account. The doctor, the nurse, the patient's father and mother, and the other patients and their families are absorbed in the story of lost love and family rivalries. They shake their heads knowingly and sympathetically click their tongues or hiss, "Aie! Yes! that is the way such problems begin." The psychiatrist has forgotten about the severe constraints on his time. But after six or seven minutes, he looks at his watch, again catches the glare of the large man pacing in and out of the room, and watches as the nurse runs off to help a family calm a greatly excited paranoid schizophrenic patient who has begun to scream, "They want to kill me! Stop them! Don't let them kill me!"

The doctor intrudes into the captivating flow of the patient's story. He fires a series of questions to assess the chief symptoms and to determine if they fulfill the criteria for clinical depression, which is what her facial expression and the story of shame and loss have suggested to him. He also sees that she is extremely pale and that her neck has a fullness when she swallows. He has made a mental note to examine her pulse and blood pressure and feel her skin to see if there are other signs to indicate either anemia or thyroid disease. But the patient has begun weeping again, in great spasms of inhalation. Her father berates her. Another patient's mother tells the father, in a solicitous tone, that it is better to let his daughter weep so that the full problem will emerge and free her of her grief. Others agree. A few begin to tell of similar problems. The doctor hushes the onlookers: "If you keep talking, I will not be able to get to you today." He begins to do a cursory physical exam. But at the same time he asks the patient to finish her story.

Sobs explode. She reaches the dénouement. Her father, who can no longer restrain himself, vehemently interjects. He disagrees with her conclusion, even with the details. He wants to retell the story. His wife tugs at his arm, whispering to him to calm himself and to let the doctor decide what is wrong. But the father is insistent. The psychiatrist responds with frustration: "If you keep interfering, how can I be of help? Which story is right, yours or hers?" Now father and daughter are arguing. Then the mother turns to the doctor and begins her own commentary; the doctor and mother continue to discuss details of the problem, until both father and daughter break in challenging her account. The psychiatrist tries to silence the parties before him, but they are now into a feud that has preoccupied their family for months. [George Bernanos (1986) wrote in his *The Diary of a Country Priest*, "Of all hate domestic hate is the most dangerous, it assuages itself by perpetual conflict, it is like open abscesses without fever which slowly poison" (p. 162).] The psychiatrist looks around with a helpless shrug. Others are commenting on the problem, some arguing different sides of the case. The large man is glaring at the psychiatrist, and shouts, "Must I wait all day? Do you not know I am a busy man?"

The psychiatrist's voice is now loud. He silences the family and the others in the room. He begins writing a prescription for an antidepressant drug. He wants the patient to come back later so that he can talk with her at greater length. The father objects. They are 25 kilometers from home and the bus leaves in half an hour.

The patient, speaking rapidly, now adds important new information. The psychiatrist first looks up impatiently, then he sits back and listens. He is shifting his diagnosis; different ideas cross his mind. He recognizes a pattern that goes beyond the disease itself and implicates a causal web of problems that he has seen many times. The differential diagnosis and the treatment for a brief moment are no longer the focus of his thoughts; rather, he visualizes a form, a set of relationships. He begins to recall the details of a case he saw last week, and one two weeks before. He sees for an instant a grand design, an integration of all the elements—the poverty, the poor housing, the inadequate diet, the endemic malaria, the parents' worries about marrying off an elder daughter and the daughter's desire for further education, the conflict over choice of a future husband, the kinship intrigues, dowry and bride price disputes, and all of a sudden it seems clear. Ah! He thinks, If only I had time to look into this question. This is where my experience shows me something that is not in our foreign textbooks. Why, of course, it is all a matter of. . . . But the illuminating thought is driven away by a nagging worry, worry about the time, all the new patients remaining to be seen, including the threatening hypomanic man, and the proper treatment for the young woman sitting before him. Yet he continues to be absorbed by the story, empathizing with the pathos of a life vulnerable and wounded in a way that he knows is ubiquitous among young women in the community.

His interest in her account shifts again. Now it is not the shared social situation, but rather the patient's unique personality and what is special in her biography that holds his attention. Why has this patient come, when so many others share the same misery? Why now? He smiles when he hears of the local remedies they have used, the rituals they have enacted, and the folk healer they have consulted. "Yes, he is a great healer. What did he say was wrong?" Yes, he thinks to himself, diet is important. That healer is a wise old fox. Imbalance in the body's constituents with an excess of cold elements does affect women. Couldn't it be a kind of metaphor of her psychophysiological vulnerability? Cold is a symbol in our classics, he muses, a sign of lost love, emptiness. . . .

All of a sudden his reverie is shattered. "Doctor! Doctor!" insinuates the nurse, whispering at his side, "Doctor, there are four new patients remaining and six return patients. Two are excited and require injections." The psychiatrist is now torn. He is into this case and wants to bring it to a proper conclusion. ["And this woman standing as though to be judged by me, had doubtless lived . . . in that horrible quietness of the desolate which of all forms of despair is the most atrocious, the most incurable, the least human . . ." (Bernanos, 1986, p. 6).] But he must move on to see the other cases. His time, his labor are the clinic's chief resources. There is so much else to do, so many others to see. This patient's gain in attention represents other patients' loss. And he has not even asked about a history of thyroid disease, the doctor realizes as he begins writing out a new prescription.

It is at this precise moment in the recurrent image that the Third World challenge to psychiatry and the opportunities and constraints on a culturally informed psychiatry meet (see Higginbotham 1983; Conors 1982; Salan and Maretzki 1984). Because here is where culture becomes unavoidable, yet psychiatry begins to shut the door. Anthropology offers concepts and a method to systematically describe the cultural patterns and relationships that intrigue the psychiatrist because he cannot but identify their importance in the causation of psychiatric conditions. He also sees that these cultural reticulations of meanings and behavioral norms affect the treatment expectations of his patients so considerably that they can be said without exaggeration to be the chief factor determining when patients get to him, whether they choose to return, and to what degree they will follow his treatment recommendations. The anthropological vision also can aid the psychiatrist in moving back and forth between the perspectives of the patient, the family, the cultural chorus of onlookers, and his own medical models.

Psychiatric knowledge, he knows all too well, is alien in this indigenous setting; hence much of his effort has to go into transforming psychiatric concepts into pragmatic explanations and treatment strategies that are culturally acceptable. Even the psychiatrist's understanding of the greater (informal) health care system in which he practices—including self and family care, folk healers and non-biomedical professionals—and the significance for his patients of alternative healers and therapies benefits from a marriage of anthropology with psychiatry. I believe that throughout much of the world, the psychiatric orientation is initially welcoming to this complementary perspective. But under the enormous pressure of having to act therapeutically in exigent circumstances with too little time, too few material resources, too limited information, and with the expectation that drugs will be the major therapeutic modality, the psychiatrist withdraws from the ethnographic account. He may even feel threatened by it. For while he will recognize that ethnography and social analysis of the biographical narrative provide information crucial for the care of individual patients and also essential to understand the community's needs, the psychiatrist experiences their potential to delay diagnosis and treatment, to turn attention from psychopathology to social pathology, over which his training leads him to believe he can exert limited if any control, and thereby to interrupt the efficient (bureaucratic) management of cases.

What is the psychiatrist to do? The usual answer is that he must be trained to expeditiously apply clinical algorithms that assure an accurate disease diagnosis and the appropriate use of somatic therapies, especially drugs and ECT. The argument is then made that he has no time to attend to the patient's story. That should be the work of the folk healer or, if there are any, the local representatives of social welfare agencies. In my experience, if this is what the psychiatrist in a non-Western setting ends up doing, i.e., treating disease but not illness, we can be sure of several things. Over time he will have a high likelihood of fashioning a kind of care that is veterinary, that is not respectful of the humanity of his patients or even of simple medical ethics, that is inattentive to prevention, and that fails to help the patient and family with their most significant concern: managing the experience of illness (see Kleinman 1980; Weisberg and Long, eds., 1984; Higginbotham 1984). This kind of care, he will lament, empowers no one, neither the patient nor the healer. Furthermore, interviews with psychiatrists in rural areas of the Third World convince me that in a few years time, he will seek to leave this practice, which he will feel dehumanizes him along with his patients.

The alternative is the tremendous challenge to create a combined clinical methodology that fosters both the treatment of disease and the interpretation of illness meanings. To accomplish this objective requires transformation of the structure of delivering care as much as the care itself. The challenge is to develop both a clinical methodology to facilitate the mini-ethnography and other of the anthropological strategies I have described in the preceding chapter, and a model for the delivery system that will provide the psychiatrist with the necessary time, space, and other resources. The former is a professional issue, the latter a political one. Without the former, the psychiatrist applies Western categories that frequently have limited relevance to his cases (cf. Connor 1982; Mullings 1985; Gaines and Farmer 1986). The development of an Indian, Chinese, or Indonesian psychiatry is unlikely without such a culturally informed methodology. To implement that clinical approach, however, will require political and economic, as much as professional, change. There is already evidence from community health care programs that such change can occur (see Lumsden, ed., 1984)—e.g., empowering communities through the transfer of knowledge and technical resources, extension of services from agencies to family and work settings, development of mental health programs in schools, in refugee camps, and for high-risk groups such as teenage mothers—though it is difficult and consuming of time and of other even more limited resources.

But how can a culturally informed methodology be implemented by a Third World psychiatrist under today's conditions or those realistically likely to be available by the end of this century? Again I ask, what is the psychiatrist to do? Does he give up "Western" diagnoses and treatments? With the best of intentions, a naive application of anthropological objectives could produce the worst of results by removing from the clinician the few tools that allow him to be effective, while stimulating his interest in activities for which he has no mandate, no resources, and no training. Does the psychiatrist struggle to fashion a five-minute ethnography (an oxymoron if there was one)? Does he become a community change agent instead of a clinician? The implication of the case vignette would seem to be that a major family or community intervention is needed. But neither the family nor the community have sought it. Perhaps they would not tolerate such an intervention, even if resources could be scraped together to launch one.

However, there are practical things that can be done. To begin with, the psychiatrist is unlikely to see this patient and her family members on only one occasion. They may return. Thus, he can organize his evaluation and treatment over a number of sessions. This makes more feasible the step-by-step assembly of a mini-ethnography. That descriptive account also is made possible by the psychiatrist's existing knowledge of the local social system and of the pertinent problems of many other patients whom he has treated. Because this patient's problem is one she shares with many others, it is wholly appropriate for the psychiatrist to become engaged with the community. Indeed, in rural settings in non-Western societies, it is almost impossible for the psychiatrist to avoid such engagement. He holds high status in the community. Thus, he interacts with local and also regional leaders. His advice is sought on many matters; his connections with other physicians, teachers, religious leaders, heads of villages and of extended families, perhaps even those from the very village from which this patient comes, are extensive. Furthermore, his clinic is quite probably part of integrated primary care services that have community development and preventive programs. Social development has become so salient an issue to health programs supported by WHO, the World Bank, the United Nations Development Program, AID and its European equivalents, the major private foundations interested in international health, and Third World nations themselves that quite possibly his region already has a demonstration project which links health care to social change activities. Although national agencies and regional officials in developing societies will differ on how appropriate they regard an individual psychiatrist's community activities to be, he is not a private practitioner, but part of the public sector, and as a result, his local responsibilities will normally include development of outreach and follow-up programs. Hence his mandate usually can be broadened to encompass all sorts of community activities on behalf of the sick and their families.

Funding, technical resources, and physician manpower, of course, will be quite limited. But this psychiatrist may have access to a surprisingly large number of paraprofessional, health education, and community agency personnel. Therefore, it may be feasible for him to implement at least several innovations in the delivery of psychiatric care. He may be able to supervise other members of the health team (e.g., a public health nurse or a social worker or a health education or nutrition student) who can visit the patient's home to undertake a limited family or neighborhood intervention. The psychiatrist can also assist nurse practitioners, primary care physicians, and public health aides, who routinely see patients with significant psychosocial problems, in deploying a broader array of family and social network interventions. Finally, the numbers of social scientists (usually at B.A. or M.A. level) are increasing rapidly in non-Western, especially Asian, societies. It may not be out of the question for the psychiatrist to have access to a social scientist or a social science student who can assist in teaching clinic staff culturally relevant topics, or in improving communication with patients. That individual may also make it feasible for the psychiatrist to collect baseline social survey and epidemiological data, and even to initiate a small research project aimed at developing highly focused sociotherapeutic and preventive interventions, such as self-help groups, social support for at-risk populations (e.g., unemployed adolescents), advocacy for community programs, training of lay therapists, and so forth.

It is unclear how many of these activities a particular practitioner will be able to undertake. Substantial change in the system of delivering care is not often in the cards. But usually there is room to make a few more limited changes. One or two anthropological strategies may be feasible, if the psychiatrist is made aware of them and if he has some interest in trying them out. For most family and personal problems, radical change is unnecessary, and may even be counterproductive. Often a modest effect is all that is required to give the protagonists time to gain purchase on a dilemma and agree on a face-saving compromise. Simply witnessing the story of an intimate conflict may encourage the warring parties to reconsider and reconcile. Even if it doesn't have this effect, listening to their accounts may suggest how leverage can be used to reconstitute family loyalties and repair marital or parental relationships. If properly prepared to define and respond to such quotidian dramas, the psychiatrist can exert a therapeutic effect that is amplified well beyond his small clinic and few staff. To be practically useful, his preparation must draw on anthropologically informed knowledge of local crises and culturally appropriate interventions, of local resources and how they can be mobilized, of the indigenous version of practical wisdom about human affairs.

Let us leave this first image, uncertain of what can and will happen in the future. In the year 2000, more than 80 percent of the world's population will live in non-Western societies. The three nations from which I have assembled this picture of Third World psychiatry—China, India, and Indonesia—will together comprise more than 40 percent of all men and women. A similarly high percentage of the world's burden of psychiatric disorders and mental health conditions (e.g., schizophrenia, depression, and anxiety disorders, organic brain syndromes caused by tropical diseases, developmental problems due to malnutrition and repeated childhood infections, substance abuse and the violence it engenders, adolescent suicide, dementia among the aged, traumas of forced uprooting and family breakdown) will be found in these societies. Will the attitudes, knowledge, and skills of the psychiatrists in these and the other non-Western societies remain Western-oriented, as they are today? If so, can psychiatry ever be anything but alien and marginal to most of the world's psychiatric patients? As these nations modernize well into the twenty-first century, will psychiatry be part of that immense process of transformation? If so, can it usefully indigenize, creating effective cultural variants without drawing on anthropological knowledge? Again if so, will not these culturally authorized psychiatric systems (e.g., an Indian or Chinese psychiatry) recursively influence psychiatry in the West? (Perhaps they will do so by clarifying which aspects of professional knowledge are culture-bound and by innovating new forms of psychiatric practice.) Can psychiatry claim to be a universal science if it fails to address the questions of its non-Western practitioners? In a world as ethnically polarized as ours, can culture continue to be as peripheral to psychiatry as it currently is regarded by psychiatrists, if psychiatry is to become at all relevant to the problems of ethnic conflict, migration, and social change? It seems to me that the gist of this line of reasoning must argue for a more central confrontation of psychiatric science with the science of culture, of psychiatric research and practice with ethnography, of the psychiatric profession with the profession of anthropology.

II

In the second image, I am conducting rounds with a small group of psychiatry residents and fellows on the consultation-liaison psychiatry service in a general hospital in the United States. We are visiting the room of a patient with a medical disorder who is also suspected of suffering from a psychiatric condition. The patient is a recent Cambodian refugee (but he could as well be Haitian, Pakistani, or Nicaraguan). He does not speak English. Nor do we speak his language. A call is put in for a translator.

Within a few minutes, an attractive, well-dressed, utterly North American–looking young woman enters the room. She is, we learn, a graduate student at the university, an art history major who works part time at the hospital. She smiles at us, and we chat for a moment in English, which she speaks fluently, with an American inflection, as one would expect of someone who came to the States at age five. Her family is from the elite class of her society, she tells us. Then she turns to the patient.

He is an elderly male. Sometimes I visualize him as a member of an ethnic minority even within his own society (e.g., a Chinese Cambodian, a Hmong from Vietnam, an Afghan refugee in Pakistan, or a Mesquito Indian from Nicaragua). From a peasant family in a distant rural area, he has never lived in a large city. He speaks a local patois that is difficult for the interpreter to grasp. It is filled with earthy expressions and religious metaphors that she finds almost impossible to translate.

Based on getting to know a number of refugees and interviewing them about problems with translators, I can describe dimensions of this hypothetical patient's experience which are all too real in the thoughts and emotions of my respondents. He is deeply embarrassed (in keeping with his culture's conventions) to be discussing such private problems with a stranger, and one of a different generation and of the opposite sex too. He is greatly self-conscious that he is speaking to someone whose tones and formal grammar show her to be from the upper class. From her dress and accent, he gathers that she is already a "foreigner," one of them. How to respond to her prying questions? How to tell her of his sadness for the homeland? How to explain the meaning of giving up the land? The shame of having left the ancestral graves unattended. The desperate loneliness of having parted from the graves of his parents, his brothers, and his wife. The immense need to return home to die. She is like his grandchildren, whom he would never talk to about these things. It is unheard of among his people for an old man to ask the help of a young woman. Why, she probably doesn't even know the songs I feel I must sing to honor the dead, he laments to himself. She would laugh at him, he knows from experience, if he told her that he must find a spirit-medium to propitiate the ancestral shades and learn which one is attacking him. What does she know of the hunger of ghosts if they are not fed by their oldest living descendants, he broods as he listens to her questions? Clearly, she is too American to believe in the old religion. Why look, he thinks, she even wears shamelessly a Christian cross around her neck.

We have requested the interpreter to ask the patient if he hears voices when no one else is in the room. She and he then begin a discussion that lasts several minutes. "I don't think he hears voices," she tells us. "What do you mean? What did you talk about with him for so long?" "He told me that he sometimes hears the ancestors weeping. I think he is from an old-fashioned background. This is a way peasants have of speaking. He doesn't really mean he hears crying. I have told him not to speak such superstitious stuff, because he is in America now."*

---

*I have recorded exchanges like this at least ten times in observations of translators working with refugee patients and Caucasian physicians.

This well-intentioned translator has just made it extremely unlikely that the patient will tell her anything that really matters to him. She has made it clear that she is alienated from the traditional culture. She is sensitive enough, however, not to mistake the normative imagery of crying ancestors for the pathological symptom hallucination. Others I have worked with might well have turned that expression into a sign of psychosis. But most translators, in my experience, indicate in subtle or not so subtle ways to the patient exactly what she has shown him—namely, that the hold of tradition has broken for them; that they do not want to hear and especially do not want the psychiatrists to hear about traditional beliefs and behaviors; and that they can no longer empathically understand the ancient idioms and archaic rhythms of a radically different way of life.

Anthropologically informed psychiatric practice calls for an entirely different kind of interpretation: an ethnographic hermeneutics that seeks to describe the patient's words in their native context of meaning and that searches for the self among its cultural imagery. That style of translation indicates the difficulty of translating from the indigenous language into English and vice versa. The anthropologically informed translator and psychiatrist are concerned not just with lexical matters but with semantics, semiotics and the interpretation of distinctive perceptual, cognitive and affective processes. Like the art historian and literacy critic, they wish to understand the meaning of symbolic forms; both in the terms of the forms themselves and in those of the mental health discourse.

This image can be extended to patients of the same culture as the psychiatrist's, but of different regional backgrounds and social statuses. Their experiences of illness may require a similar kind of anthropologically informed translation. Here many of the constraints on psychiatric practice in the Third World, described in the first image, may also affect psychiatrists in our own and other industrialized societies. The same obstacles and opportunities surround this challenge to conventional professional practice. In the sense that I am now describing, each psychiatric interview can be analogized to translation across distinctive languages and cultures—i.e., the idiom and conventions of medicine and those of the popular culture (see Mishler 1984). I believe many psychiatrists will accept the image, but few will be willing to agree, in my experience, that such ethnographic translation requires special knowledge and skills. That is to say, psychiatrists conduct informal ethnographies and phenomenological interpretations without being trained in the key concepts and methods of translation. Some succeed expertly; some do not; and many who could work much more effectively with patients never rigorously engage the conceptual basis for doing so.

There is a systematic approach to cross-cultural and cross-ethnic patient-doctor encounters that begins with the techniques to develop trust and rapport, then moves on to the formal elicitation of symptom complaints and explanatory models in their literal wording. In the next stage, the practitioner employs the translator and family members as key informants to provide a figurative interpretation of the patient's statements (and also what is implied by silence and nonverbal communication) in light of their cultural significance and also their idiosyncratic importance to the patient. Then the practitioner draws on this insider's knowledge to reformulate questions that clarify the diagnosis and complete the patient's narrative. There are specific ways of checking the validity of the interpreter's account and detecting characteristic problems of cross-cultural miscommunication, including use of the same word to mean different things and of different words to signify the same thing. Culture-blind spots, created by regional, ethnic, class, gender, and age differences, can also be systematically assessed. The translation of the practitioner's explanatory model and the process of negotiation with the patient's (and family's) model can be organized within a standard framework that avoids common pitfalls. Such culturally informed frameworks, which are outlined in a number of useful publications for practitioners, not only improve translation but often exert a direct therapeutic effect (see Harwood, ed., 1981; E. H. B. Lin 1984; Katon and Kleinman 1981; Rosen and Kleinman 1984; Johnson and Kleinman 1984 and in press). For example, the translator can be trained by the psychiatrist or others to act as a culture broker who assists the patient and family to accommodate to hospital and clinic rules and professional and societal norms that are frequently alien, and for that reason threatening and alienating to patients who are refugees or recent immigrants (Kaufert et al. 1985; Weidman 1978:819–56; Tripp-Reimer and Brink 1985). Such cultural brokerage, fostered by the informed empathy of the psychiatrist, can, in my experience, fairly rapidly remoralize patients. A culturally oriented psychiatric assessment will also look for common problems that occur at particular points in the acculturation process—e.g., expectable early depression and anxiety, transient paranoid states, later-occurring and more serious forms of pathology; it will also organize care, including supportive psychotherapy, in culturally consonant ways. Tseng, McDermott, and Maretzki (1974), among others, have established techniques for providing psychotherapy tailored to the expectations and needs of particular ethnic groups. While controlled, double-blind clinical trials have not been conducted to evaluate the efficacy of such culturally oriented therapy, it is the impression of many therapists that this can be a therapeutically effective practice to relieve suffering and influence the quality of life for many refugees, recent immigrants, and even for numbers of established ethnic minorities. The formulation of the mini-ethnography should assist the practitioner to pinpoint culturally salient problems—e.g., the unique family-based stigma of serious mental illness among Chinese and its tendency to encourage predictable kinds of problems in help seeking, compliance, and long-term care (T. Y. Lin and M. C. Lin 1982)—and to provide appropriate treatment strategies to respond to these problems. Other examples could be given of how the systemization of cultural awareness and the application of culturally informed treatment interventions empower the psychiatrist to provide better care for his patients and their family members (Gaw, ed., 1982; McGoldrick et al., eds., 1982; Tseng, McDermott and Maretzki 1974).

An additional major task for all physicians, which is acquiring special importance in our times, is translating between the increasingly complex concepts of medical science and the lay understanding of risk and disorder and treatment by members of the popular culture. As a patient of mine once put it, "We none of us know what to make of risks anymore. We've been told too many different things. If you be just an ordinary person how can you figure it? What do you eat? What don't you? The world looks so bloody dangerous. Who can say what caused it, my cancer. And the treatment, Doc. I'm only a high school graduate. I can't even understand the simplified explanations" (Kleinman 1988).

There is no training for physicians in translating from the language of medical science to the language of patients and families. We usually think of this as a problem facing high-technology tertiary-care specialists. But in fact every physician confronts this interpretive gap. Psychiatrists will increasingly be called on to help their patients understand genetics, immunology, neuroscience, and more, and to correct the erroneous pictures provided by the media, which claim much more is known than in fact is and that much more can be clinically applied than in fact can be. Again an anthropologically sophisticated approach to this problem goes well beyond simple awareness, i.e., "sensitivity," by modeling it as a series of predictable (and remediable) miscommunications in translation between different modes of knowledge and ways of knowing (professional and lay cultures'), not simply a question of the provision of health education. A cultural perspective shows that this problem is a major obstacle to efficient health education about vaccination, appropriate use of primary care facilities, and mental health and other public health programs, especially in the Third World but also in the most technologically advanced societies. Whether such a model of cultural translation can be usefully applied in the context of practical patient care is yet another test in the development of a culturally informed psychiatry.

III

The third image is a composite, a montage assembled from field observations in a variety of different professional settings where formal knowledge is created and applied. In one component, we are in a North American epidemiological research unit, observing a research team "clean" and "code" data from questionnaires used in a community survey. The team is experiencing difficulty deciding on the data "reduction" from an interview with the depressed owner of a small family business in the deteriorating section of the city.

"Is he or isn't he anhedonic?"

"Well, he says that he still has the same old interests—fishing and golfing and reading—but they are not quite the same as before. He says, 'They are pleasurable, but they are not quite the same as before.'"

"Did he say anything else?"

"Nothing else is recorded, but I remember him. I observed part of the interview. Isn't he the one who said that he used to love to eat the pan-fried trout he caught, but they didn't have the same taste anymore? That sounds like anhedonia to me."

"Wait a minute gentlemen, you know the rule. Unless it is written on the questionnaire, or in your daily diary, or has been tape-recorded, it doesn't count. We do that to protect against just this kind of bias. Remember?"

"OK, how do we score it then? Do we say he isn't anhedonic, and disregard what Doug remembers? We can't go back to him. And even if we could, it wouldn't reflect the time the interview was completed."

"It's a big decision here. This guy doesn't report sadness or depressed feelings or even irritability. But he gives six vegetative complaints and looked depressed to the interviewer. If we don't score it 'anhedonia,' we can't diagnose him as a case of major depressive disorder. So?"

Another component of this combined image is a scene from a meeting of the mental health team in a small health maintenance organization on the West Coast. Present are two psychiatrists, two clinical psychologists, a group of social workers, and an administrator.

Administrator: "Here's a problem! Too many hospitalizations last month. Keep this up and we'll break the bank. Are you sure we need to put so many people in the hospital?"

Psychologist: "You should see the patients we are not admitting (*to the hospital*). There are some pretty sick people. We are keeping psychotic patients, even a few people who could easily become suicidal, in the clinic."

Administrator: "Well, I'm just telling you the problem. We need to find a solution."

Psychiatrist: "Maybe the solution is that we need more resources. More professional staff, and more funds to hospitalize people."

Administrator: "All right. If we can't be serious about this, we may have to live with consequences that affect us all and the viability of the program."

We are in the office of a disability agency. A pending chronic pain case is being discussed by a lay examiner and a consulting psychiatrist. I paraphrase their discussion.

Examiner: OK, she is in a fair amount of pain, and it makes her anxious, but so are a lot of people. There are no listings for pain.* If she is to be determined disabled, you know as well as I do, she must make a listing. She needs a medical or mental diagnosis.

Psychiatrist: She is disabled. I feel there is no question of her functional impairment. Yet she doesn't make the mental listings. Her problem is pain, not a psychiatric disorder. But if I'm pushed to the wall, I think I could justify the diagnosis of a chronic anxiety disorder. Even though the anxiety is the consequence, not the cause, of her disability.

Examiner: If that is the way you read it, it makes sense to me. I mean she is seriously impaired. But we've got a problem with the bureaucratic regs.

A final part of the composite image comes from a meeting of a research review committee of a mental health funding agency. The committee has just heard the main reviewers of a grant proposal split over whether it should be funded or not. I paraphrase the ensuing discussion.

Chairman: We have got a problem. We need to come to a decision to approve at a priority too high to fund or at a fundable score. *(Priority scores range from 1 to 5, with 1 as the most fundable score.)*

Member: There are a lot of issues here. Given the split over the scientific quality of the proposal, I wonder if we can't decide on the basis of the scientific value of this kind of research. I'm not an expert in this field, but I think it is of less scientific significance than other approaches to this problem in psychiatry today.

Reviewer 1: That is a difficult thing to prove. I am persuaded by

---

In order to be awarded disability benefits from the Social Security Administration, a patient must have a specific medical or psychiatric condition "listed" on an official agency taxonomy of conditions warranting the label "disabled." Pain, which is supposed to be "taken into account" in the evaluation process, does not in and of itself qualify as a disabling condition. Since the patient under discussion, like most chronic pain patients, does not have a clear-cut medical disorder which is directly responsible for the pain, the evaluation team must find a pertinent psychiatric listing or deny the patient's claim.

the authors that this is an important approach. Granted it is not the "in" way to study this problem. So what!

Reviewer 2: Hold on! These are the only guys doing this kind of thing. The approach is a dead end. People are now doing . . .

Chairman: Do we have a paradigm conflict? It sounds awfully like one.

Member: I don't agree. I think there is room for honest disagreement over which approaches to a psychiatric problem are scientifically sounder and more useful.

Member: How do you determine that from what is the popular bandwagon of the moment? Everyone jumps on board new bandwagons of technically more sophisticated research designs and data-analytic tools. Plenty of fine work has been done by scholars working outside the mainstream scientific approach, or even going against it. No one has invalidated their methodology.

Chairman: Is there a proposal we can vote on, or do we want more time to discuss the details?

Let these four components serve to project a montage of psychiatry in various bureaucratic settings—research unit, HMO, disability agency, research review committee. I could have included other scenes—e.g., psychiatrist in the courtroom; expert testimony to a local or national governmental committee; an insurance company's committee providing psychiatric review of quality and cost of care; psychiatrists in the school system; committees to organize psychiatric teaching in medical schools. Each of those settings would, I think, contribute to a similar composite image. That image discloses that psychiatry is part of the bureaucratic structure of contemporary Western society, and within that structure it is routinely involved in *negotiations* over the application of professional knowledge to practical problems. Those negotiations affect clinical judgment, diagnostic decisions, bureaucratic standards, institutional goals, even the science of psychiatry. That is to say, practice and teaching and research are part of elaborate social structures where psychiatric knowledge is socially created and its application transacted. Psychiatry, like the rest of medicine and the other professions, cannot be understood apart from its bureaucratic settings and their political, financial, and institutional constraints.

Taken together, the four images make the case for a much more serious consideration of *culture* in the science and practice of psychiatry. They also suggest that over the long run the profession will find social analysis of increasing pertinence, perhaps even unavoidable.

Of all the medical specialties, I contend, psychiatry has the most pervasive relationship to culture. Psychiatry is, to begin with, a window on a culture's sources of distress and on the human consequences of such distress. While certain psychiatric conditions (e.g., schizophrenia, manic-depressive psychosis, major depressive disorder, and organic brain syndromes) would qualify as *disease* in virtually any nosologic system, other psychiatric conditions (e.g., the personality disorders, low-grade depressive and anxiety experiences, various marital, family, and school crises, perhaps many of the so-called culture-bound syndromes) may be assigned a medical label in one era or society but may be just as compellingly regarded as religious or moral problems or simply as perturbations in the social fabric of daily living in other times and places. The latter are so thoroughly cultural judgments that major transformations in a society's values will determine whether they are called disease, sin, or crime (e.g., consider the history of substance abuse in the West). Still other psychiatric conditions—e.g., post-traumatic stress syndromes following wars or revolutions, depression caused by forced uprooting and acculturation, antisocial behavior among unemployed adolescents in urban slums—are the very stuff of those societal transformations. The psychiatrist experiences, moreover, in his own professional identity the fears and stigma that attach to serious mental illness. His diagnostic criteria are infiltrated with cultural norms and biases. His treatment is founded on the very apparatus of culture—words, symbols, meanings, not least of all his own social persona and charisma. The ethical commitments of his practice are constrained by cultural values. (One must also acknowledge that culture is influential in the rest of medicine, but not nearly to the same extent as in psychiatry).

To rethink psychiatry from a cross-cultural perspective, then, is to confront culture itself. How we think of culture will strongly influence how we configure the relationship between psychiatry and its cultural context.

I write these concluding words with modest expectation. I point toward no apocalypse. I call for no revolution.* I have no ultimate answers. I recognize my perspective is at the margin, not the center, of psychiatry; but I do not accept that the questions I have posed represent too extreme a point of view. Because I am a practicing psychiatrist, I am well aware of the extraordinary pressures that my profession and my colleagues are experiencing. The profession of psychiatry, like the profession of medicine of which it is part, is in the throes of a great social change that is affecting many other institutions and individuals in these times and that is making

---

In fact, I would argue that carefully controlled efforts at limited, focused change in the vicious cycles within local social systems, e.g., those which conduce to mental illness or others which impede the effective delivery of humane care—with all the uncertainty and ad hoc character such efforts entail—offer the most promising prospect for being of help. Together with key policy changes, sharply defined local social interventions offer a practical and more human focus for psychiatry. (See Moore 1987 for a somewhat similar view of efforts at controlling the more menacing effects of authority and inequality.)

the world a different place. Practice grows more complex. Our problems are more confusing. Great issues—particularly economic and medical-legal—swirl around us, only a few of which are covered in these pages.

I know that social factors are not the sole determinants of mental disorders. Genetic sources of vulnerability must not be discounted because from a naive perspective they seem to threaten liberal political values any more than environmental sources of risk can be avoided because they seem to challenge conservative philosophy (Jencks 1987). Biological advances are of great significance to psychiatry, as are new developments in our understandings of the self and its inner workings. An effective integration of the biological, the psychological, and the social is not around the corner. In spite of that, patients come to the psychiatrist for solutions. They want us to do something to help them. Care is exigent and difficult at the best of times. And I think many will agree these are not the best of times.

Antipsychiatry critics are dangerously irresponsible: mental illness is real; most psychiatrists neither misuse nor abuse psychiatry. Psychiatry is of increasing value to patients and their families. I have always counted it a privilege to be a psychiatrist. I continue to be optimistic about the role psychiatry can play to alleviate suffering and assure that health care is responsive to the human dimensions of illness. I am for psychiatry.

I am also realistic about what is feasible to accomplish. The cultural perspective is not going to become the central paradigm of the psychiatric profession, at least not in my lifetime. Nor does it hold the answers to all of the many serious problems besetting the discipline. Yet I continue to believe the questions I have asked of the profession can no longer be avoided or regarded as peripheral. They touch the very essence of what it is to be part of psychiatry in this period of difficult transition from a twentieth century that has been largely dominated by Western concerns and elite-class perspectives to a twenty-first century that is virtually certain to be much more substantially focused on the concerns and perspectives of the non-Western world and that is also likely to give priority to the interests of a much wider range of the world's population including the poor. If psychiatrists turn away from the central questions raised in this and the preceding chapters, and the many subsidiary issues they contain, we can be sure that governments, other health and social welfare disciplines, and laymen and women will not.

Take, for example, psychiatry's disappointingly marginal place in international health institutions and programs. This failure of the profession represents, in large measure, a lack of interest among the Western professionals who have dominated psychiatry from its origin. The rapid development of psychiatric services in the Third World is changing the on-the-ground reality. Whether or not psychiatrists in the developed societies gain a serious interest in the problems faced by their colleagues in the Third World, who are fashioning new approaches to remake psychiatric diagnoses and treatments so that they are more appropriate to the pressing problems of poor non-Western populations, those colleagues will be exerting an influence on international health bodies and programs. That influence may well come to shape the debate on international mental health policy, much as is happening in the rest of the health field. Theory and research will also feel this shift in priorities. By the end of the century or not long thereafter, the orientation of the psychiatric profession as a whole, which from its origin has been centered on issues of importance to the West, will, like the broader field of medicine and public health, swing toward a more balanced position vis-à-vis the burden of morbidity in the developing world, where most psychiatric patients and, perhaps sooner than has been predicted, most psychiatrists will be found. At that point, a Western-oriented profession that has taken a serious interest in the cultural questions reviewed in these chapters will be in a far more enlightened position to respond to the international challenge to its priorities. Much the same kind of analysis could be written about the important implications for psychiatry of the increasing numbers of refugees and ethnic minorities and the increasing salience of ethnic conflicts and their mental health consequences around the globe.

For these external reasons as much as because of the internal dynamics of change that I have just charted at work at present within the profession, the cultural program in one form or another is sure to receive over time much greater attention at all levels of the profession of psychiatry and of the other mental health professions. When that has come about, regardless of the advances in biological understanding (which we can only hope will be considerable), we will look backward toward this period either as a continuation of powerful professional resistance to the coming crisis in our priorities or as the beginning of the transition toward a global psychiatry whose science and practices accommodate an international mental health agenda, cross-cultural differences, the social context, and, not least of all, the social sciences.

Notes

Prologue (pp. 1–4)

1. There are, of course, other anthropological visions. A radical culturalist account of mental illness holds that schizophrenia and other mental disorders are solely categories in Western culture. These cultural categories create normal experience and constitute abnormality too. The radical culturalist viewpoint includes a role for politicoeconomic forces as the sources of authority and inequality that, it is claimed, are reproduced in mental disorder and its treatment (Foucault 1966). But culturalists are strangely quiet about experience and its psychobiological roots, about why some become mentally ill but most do not.

   Schizophrenia, for example, is said to be inseparable from the Western concept of a bounded self. It is said to be constituted out of the menacing cultural preoccupation that the self can be split apart (Barrett, in press). That metaphor of the divided self, it is claimed, reproduces the constraints of Western capitalist social formations in the person.

   While important insights inform this vision, it ascribes to cultural meanings such enormous power that there is little but culture to deal with. Culture, so defined, becomes a total system, a vast and amorphous explanatory paradigm that explains everything—and thus nothing. There is no way that it can be operationalized. The radical culturalist interpretation cannot adequately deal with similar mental disorders that occur in greatly different cultures, or other issues crucial to the understanding of mental disorder on the level of the sick person, the family, and the practitioner.

   There is also a radical materialist view which, like the dominant explanatory paradigm in psychiatry, gives primacy in the cause and effect of mental illness to biology. Here there is no place for culture, and little enough for social relations and psychology. The inadequacies of this positivist perspective are explored in the chapters that follow.

I find the middle ground—where culture and biology reciprocally interact—the best vantage point from which to make sense of the cross-cultural data base and to avoid the excesses of its extremist neighbors. I have elsewhere referred to this epistemological position as a cultural interactionist or modified relativist stance (see Kleinman 1986; Hahn and Kleinman 1984). When I refer to the anthropological vision, I mean this perspective.

Chapter 1 *(pp. 5–17)*

1. I have provided this patient with a pseudonym and altered a few identifying details of her life story to protect her anonymity.

2. *Shenjing shuairuo* in Chinese. For discussions of neurasthenia in China, readers can consult Kleinman (1982, 1986); Lin, Kleinman, and Lin (1982); and Lin, ed., in press.

3. China's Great Proletarian Cultural Revolution began in 1966. The initial targets of the Cultural Revolution were intellectuals. Later cadres in the Communist Party and in other institutions became targets. Eventually, virtually all Chinese were affected by the Cultural Revolution as victims or victimizers. But for intellectuals it must stand as one of the worse episodes in China's history and perhaps also in world history. Intellectuals were systematically attacked (politically, psychologically, and physically), degraded, and discriminated against. They were sent to rural areas to "learn from the peasants" and to undergo thought reform. Their children, who were labeled as one of the "five blacks" or "nine bads", were also sent to the countryside and were kept from advancing their education. The Red Guards were students and other urban youth who at first carried out the abuses on behalf of Mao Zedong and his fellow ultraleftist leaders in China. Later they too became victims. In the three worst years of the Cultural Revolution, 1966–69, tens and perhaps hundreds of thousands were killed or committed suicide. The moral fabric of Chinese society tore apart. A massive delegitimation crisis alienated many Chinese from the society's value system, creating anomie—a wounding personal sense of meaninglessness and dread and loss. The Cultural Revolution wound down in the early seventies but was not officially brought to a close until 1976. For accounts of the effect of the Cultural Revolution on the lives of intellectuals, readers can consult several deeply moving personal accounts (Liang and Shapiro 1983; Yue and Wakeman 1985; Cheng 1987) and one outstanding overview (Thurston 1987). I report other, more detailed case histories of the psychiatric victims of the Cultural Revolution in Kleinman (1986).

4. Members of China's "lost generation" of students whose education was interrupted by the Cultural Revolution have found it extremely difficult to gain admission to university, one of the few avenues of social mobility. During the Cultural Revolution many were denied admission on political grounds. Afterward they had to compete against the much better prepared next generation of students. Inasmuch as 5 percent or fewer pass the rigorous entrance examination, repeated failure is a shared experience for many members of the lost generation. Feelings of desperate shame are common, for these are the children of intellectuals who feel that they have failed their parents and their tradition as well as themselves.

5. See Staiano's (1986) excellent review of the semiotics of illness diagnoses, and my commentary on it and the theory of illness meaning (Kleinman 1987).

6. Segments of this section are adapted from Kleinman 1987.

7. As Asaad and Shapiro (1986) conclude in a recent "state of the art" review of hallucinations, psychiatrists regard hallucinations as important signs of pathology. When they are part of a normal experience, Asaad and Shapiro suggest they be called "pseudo-hallucinations"—a sensibility I believe most psychiatrists share.

8. Of the large literature on neurasthenia, the following sources are particularly useful: Beard (1891); Chatel and Peele (1971); Drinka (1984); Lin, ed. (in press); Rosenberg (1962); Sicherman (1977).

Chapter 2 (pp. 18–33)

1. Sections of this chapter are adapted and expanded from Kleinman (1987). The review of the methodological issues benefited greatly from collaboration with Professors Peter Guarnaccia and Byron Good.

2. An interesting collection of illustrations of the value of combining anthropological and epidemiological methods can be found in Janes et al. (1986). That volume should convince even diehard defenders of ethnography that it can be combined with quantitative epidemiological techniques to the benefit of both disciplines.

Chapter 3 (pp. 34–52)

1. The genetic theory of schizophrenia, which up until several years ago seemed well established, is now in considerable disarray. Inheritance has not been proved (see Barnes 1987a). There is evidence of abnormalities in dopamine receptors in key regions of the brain. The response of patients to antipsychotic drugs also points to dopamine neurotransmission as disordered. But other biological findings are controversial (e.g., alleged altered brain blood flow and larger ventricles). There is still, after more than 30 years of intensive biological investigation, no clear-cut understanding of the biology of schizophrenia (Haracz 1982; Lewontin, Kamin and Rose 1984; Barrett in press). This does not deter psychiatrists and those who write the advertisements for drug companies from asserting without any hesitation that schizophrenia is a biologically based disorder. This belief is a central tenet of professional orthodoxy.

   The most convincing research on the genetics of a mental illness comes from Egeland et al. (1987), who studied bipolar (manic-depressive) disorder, which has a 0.5 to 1 percent prevalence rate in the West, among Old Order Amish in the U.S. They established that a gene or chromosome 11 is associated with dominant inheritance. But there is only partial "penetration," meaning that environmental factors are still essential in the expression of the genetic vulnerability. Other research suggests different genetic factors in other populations in which bipolar disease has been studied.

2. The topic of colonial impediments to accurate psychiatric findings from India and Africa in the nineteenth and early twentieth centuries is reviewed in Weiss and Kleinman in press.

3. The most recent Cuban migration to the U.S. did include patients with mental illness who were forced to depart for Florida. But this is not true of Vietnamese, Cambodian, Laotian, or South American refugee groups.

4. Showalter (1985) reviews evidence that the finding of greater rates of neurotic disorder among women seems to have been true as well of women in England during much of the nineteenth and twentieth century. Although her historical analysis indicates it affected women in all social classes, there is no epidemiological data to settle the issue.

5. This section of the chapter includes materials modified from a report of an NIHM contract for a Review of Cross-Cultural Studies of Depressive and Anxiety Disorders prepared by the author and his colleagues, Byron Good and Peter Guarnaccia, in May 1986.

6. One of the more impressive demonstrations of cultural differences in symptomatology of mental illness is the reports of Jilek-Aall et al. (1978) of the symptom patterns of Russian Doukhobor, Coast Salish Indian, and Mennonite patients, whom they treated in the Fraser Valley of British Columbia, Canada. These cross-cultural psychiatrists found "that while sexes could to some extent be differentiated on the basis of clinical symptoms, cultural factors came out as the more important differentiating criteria of symptom formation." For example, for the Doukhobor psychiatric patients, violent acts against property and relatively very paranoid delusions concerning legal authority and God or Devil were common. Prolonged mourning reactions, suicide attempts, identity confusion, marital maladjustment, and hallucinations of supernatural beings differentiated Canadian Indian patients from the other two ethnic groups; whereas gastrointestinal symptoms, hypochrondriasis, apathy, feelings of inadequacy and self-depreciation, guilt and fear of rejection or punishment by God, shame, sexual dysfunction, and general and phobic anxiety set Mennonite patients apart.

7. In a long-term study of manic-depressive disorder among Old Order Amish in Pennsylvania, Egeland (1986) describes how the biological bases of the disorder, group norms, and social conditions combine to form a pattern of expressing complaints that discloses just such uniformities and differences.

8. We know little about trance as a psychophysiological as opposed to a social phenomenon in different cultures. This is particularly disquieting when we realize that in 1890 William James wrote, "A comparative study of trance . . . is meanwhile of the most urgent importance for the comprehension of our nature." (James 1890, p. 373).

Chapter 4 *(pp. 53–76)*

1. Schwab (1986), a leading social epidemiologist of mental illness, shows that counter to what is often asserted, there is not a linear relationship of mental illness to class as one descends the class ladder. Rather, the lowest socioeconomic class bears a much larger burden of mental illness than the other classes. Thus, the focus of concern should be on this class, which also has by far the highest rates of medical disease and mortality (see, for example, Black 1980).

2. Leighton (1986) suggests that where psychiatric disorder has high prevalence, as in the contemporary West, psychopathology may feed back to influence the social structure negatively. Presumably, this would cyclically affect the vulnerability to mental illness so that more individuals might be at risk.

3. In contemporary China, the status of intellectual, landlord, high-ranking cadre, or bourgeoisie became a risk factor during the Cultural Revolution for serious consequences such as post-traumatic stress disorder, depression, and suicide (Kleinman 1986; Thurston 1987). This represents a fundamental political transformation of societal values. In traditional Chinese society, intellectuals and landlords were at the top of the hierarchy of class and status. In the past decade, intellectuals and professionals and a new business class have again become publicly valued.

4. The use of medical terms like "chronic viral disease" by physicians in the contemporary U.S. is often a way of providing patients with a trendy medical label that has the same effect as "neurasthenia" in China (and in nineteenth-century North America). Psychosomatic and psychiatric labels still convey undesirable meanings for many in the U.S., and the medical profession finds ways of avoiding their use with patients for whom they are unacceptable.

5. I would argue that the mental health movement of the 1960s hardly ever developed specific techniques of social prevention. Rather the rhetoric of social change was harnessed by mental health professionals to pull treatment centers into the public consciousness and federal budget. These centers gave positions, incomes, and community influence to mental health professionals, but by and large did not organize local social interventions.

Chapter 6 *(pp. 108–141)*

1. There have also been reports that the neuroleptic malignant syndrome, a dangerous and potentially lethal effect of the antipsychotic drugs which causes lead-pipe rigidity, fever, elevated blood pressure and heart rate, and rapid breathing, is much more common than previously thought (Pope et al. 1986). This is yet another disadvantage of the use of antipsychotic agents.

2. The grid described here is a major modification of one I developed earlier (see Kleinman 1980, pp. 207–208).

Chapter 7 *(pp. 142–166)*

1. Materials in this section are adapted and revised from Kleinman 1985 and 1987.

2. Too often the potential contribution of social science is unrecognized even by those in the profession with a mandate to respond to social issues. In a recent statement, the Chief, Neuropsychiatry Branch, National Institute of Mental Health and a colleague criticized the absence of scientific data pertinent to the social policy change that eventuated in the United States in the early 1960s in deinstitutionalization and subsequently the problem of the homeless mentally ill (Wyatt and De Renzo 1986). Nowhere in this discussion is social science or social science research mentioned. Rather, the dominant image for how to examine this question is the controlled clinical trial used in drug trials. Evaluation research, the major social science approach to social policy implementation, is simply not acknowledged.

3. One line of effort that is in particular need of such support is the rather remarkable though still early steps that have been taken to marry ethnographic and epidemiological methods in the development of a more sophisticated approach to the social epidemiology of mental and other disorders (cf. Janes et al. 1986).

Bibliography

Abramson, L. Y., et al.
  1978   Learned helplessness in humans. *Journal of Abnormal Psychology* 87:49–74.

Aiken, L., and D. Mechanic, eds.
  1986   *Applications of Social Science to Clinical Medicine and Health Policy.* New Brunswick, N.J.: Rutgers University Press.

Alanen, Y. O., et al.
  1986   *Toward Need-Specific Treatment of Schizophrenic Psychoses.* New York: Springer-Verlag.

American Psychiatric Association (APA) Commission on Psychotherapies
  1982   *Psychotherapy Research: Methodological and Efficacy Issues.* Washington, D.C.: APA.

American Psychiatric Association protests UN report on rights of mentally ill.
  1987   *Psychiatric News* 22(2):1, Jan. 16.

Angel, R., and P. Thoits
  1987   The impact of culture on the cognitive structure of illness. *Culture, Medicine and Psychiatry.* 11(4):465–494.

Ansari, S. A.
  1969   Symptomatology of Indian depressives. *Transactions of the All India Institute of Mental Health*, 9:1–18.

Antonovsky, A.
  1979   *Health, Stress and Coping.* San Francisco: Jossey-Bass.

Anumonge, A.
  1970   Outpatient psychiatry in a Nigerian university general hospital. *Social Psychiatry* 5:96–99.

Asaad, G., and B. Shapiro
    1986   Hallucinations: Theoretical and clinical overview. *American Journal of Psychiatry* 143:1088–1097.

Baer, H.
    1981   Prophets and advisors in black spiritual churches: Therapy, palliative, or opiate? *Culture, Medicine and Psychiatry* 5:145–170.

Balk, D.
    1983   Adolescents' grief reactions, self-concept, and perceptions following sibling death. *Journal of Youth and Adolescence* 12(2):137–161.

Bandura, A.
    1977   *Social Learning Theory*. Englewood Cliffs, N.J.: Prentice-Hall.

Bannerman, R. H., et al., eds.
    1983   *Traditional Medicine and Health Care Coverage*. Geneva: WHO.

Barnes, D. M.
    1987   Biological issues in schizophrenia. *Science* 235:430–433.

———
    1987   Mystery disease at Lake Tahoe challenges virologists and clinicians. *Science* 234:541–542.

Baron, M., et al.
    1985   Familial transmission of schizotypal and borderline personality disorders. *American Journal of Psychiatry* 142:927–934.

Barrett, R.
    In press   Schizophrenia and personhood. *Medical Anthropology Quarterly*.

Barzun, J.
    1983   *A Stroll with William James*. Chicago: University of Chicago Press, p. 235.

Bateson, G.
    1957   In B. Schaffner, ed., *Group Processes*. New York: Josiah Macy Jr. Foundation.

Bazzoui, W.
    1970   Affective disorders in Iraq. *British Journal of Psychiatry* 117:195–203.

Beard, G.
    1891   *American Nervousness*. New York: Putnam.

Beck, A. T.
    1976   *Cognitive Therapy and the Emotional Disorders*. New York: International Universities Press.

———, J. Rush, et al.
    1979   *Cognitive Therapy of Depression*. New York: Guilford.

Beeman, W.
    1985   Dimensions of dysphoria. In A. Kleinman and B. Good, eds., *Culture and Depression*. Berkeley: University of California Press; pp. 216–243.

Beiser, M.
    1985   A study of depression among traditional Africans, urban North Americans, and Southeast Asian Refugees. In A. Kleinman and B. Good,

eds., *Culture and Depression*. Berkeley: University of California Press; pp. 272–298.

———
1987   Changing time perspective and mental health among Southeast Asian refugees. *Culture, Medicine and Psychiatry*. 11(4):437–464.

———, and J. A. E. Fleming
1986   Measuring psychiatric disorder among Southeast Asian refugees. *Psychological Medicine* 16:627–639.

Beitman, B.
1983   The demographics of American psychiatrists. *American Journal of Psychotherapy* 37:37–48.

Bell, R.
1985   *Holy Anorexia*. Chicago: University of Chicago Press.

Bergin, A. E.
1975   Psychotherapy can be dangerous. *Psychology Today*, November, 96–104.

Berkman, L.
1981   Physical health and the social environment. In L. Eisenberg and A. Kleinman, eds., *The Relevance of Social Science for Medicine*. Dordrecht, Holland: D. Reidel; pp. 51–76.

Bernanos, G.
1986   *The Diary of a Country Priest*. Translated by P. Morris. New York: Carroll and Graf. (First edition 1937).

Berris, B.
1986   Chronic viral disease. *Canadian Medical Association Journal* 135: 1260–1268, December.

Binitie, A.
1975   A factor-analytical study of depression across African and European cultures. *British Journal of Psychiatry* 127:559–563.

Black, D.
1980   *Inequality in Health: A Report*. Department of Health and Social Security, London.

Blazer, D., et al.
1985   Psychiatric disorders: a rural/urban comparison. *Archives of General Psychiatry* 41:971–978.

Bleuler, M.
1978   *The Schizophrenic Disorders: Long-Term Patient and Family Studies*. New Haven, Conn.: Yale University Press.

Bloch, F.
1986   Medical scientists in the Nazi era. *Lancet* 1:375.

Bloch, S. and M. J. Lambert
1985   What price psychotherapy? *British Journal of Psychiatry* 146:95–98.

———, and P. Reddaway
1977   *Psychiatric Terror*. New York: Basic Books.

Blumhagen, D.
1982   The meaning of hypertension. In N. Chrisman and T. Maretzki, eds., *Clinically Applied Anthropology*. Dordrecht, Holland: D. Reidel; pp. 299–324.

Boffey, P.
    1986   Psychotherapy is as good as drugs in curing depression, study finds. *New York Times,* 14 May, p. 1.

Bond, M., ed.
    1986   *The Psychology of the Chinese People.* Hong Kong: Oxford University Press.

Book, J. A., et al.
    1978   Schizophrenia in a North Swedish geographical isolate 1900–1977. *Clinical Genetics* 14:373–394.

Borus, J., et al.
    1979   Psychotherapy in a goldfish bowl. *Archives of General Psychiatry* 36:187–190.

——, et al.
    1985   The offset of mental health treatment on ambulatory medical care utilization and charges. *Archives of General Psychiatry* 42:573.

Boyd, J., and M. Weissman
    1981   Epidemiology of affective disorders. *Archives of General Psychiatry* 38:1039–1046.

Boyer, L. B.
    1964   Further remarks concerning shamans and shamanism. *Israel Annals of Psychiatry* 2(2):235–237.

Brenner, M. H.
    1973   *Mental Illness and the Economy.* Cambridge, Mass.: Harvard University Press.

    1981   Importance of the economy to the nation's health. In L. Eisenberg and A. Kleinman, eds., *The Relevance of Social Science for Medicine.* Dordrecht, Holland: D. Reidel; pp. 371–396.

    1987   Economic change, alcohol consumption and heart disease mortality in nine industrialized countries. *Social Science and Medicine* 25(2):119–132.

Brenner, S. O., and L. Levi
    1987   Long-term unemployment among women in Sweden. *Social Science and Medicine* 25(2):153–161.

Brody, H.
    1977   "Persons and Placebos: Philosophical Implications of the Placebo Effect." Ph.D. dissertation, Department of Philosophy, Michigan State University.

Brown, G., et al.
    1962   Influence of family life on the course of schizophrenic illness. *British Journal of Preventive and Social Medicine* 16:55–68.

——, et al.
    1966   *Schizophrenia and Social Care.* London: Oxford University Press.

——, J. Birley, and J. K. Wing
    1972   Influence of family life on the course of schizophrenic disorders. *British Journal of Psychiatry* 121:241–258.

———, and T. Harris
1978 *The Social Origins of Depression.* New York: Free Press.

———, T. K. J. Craig, and T. Harris
1985 Depression: Disease or distress? *British Journal of Psychiatry* 197:612–622.

———, T. Harris, and A. Bifulco
1985 Long term effects of early loss of parent. In M. Rutter, et al., eds., *Young People: Developmental and Clinical Perspectives.* New York: Guilford.

———, et al.
1986 Social support, self esteem and depression. *Psychological Medicine.* 16:813–831.

Bynum, C. W.
In press Holy Anorexia in modern Portugal. *Culture, Medicine and Psychiatry.*

Cacioppa, J., and R. Petty, eds.
1983 *Social Psychophysiology.* New York: Guilford.

Canino, G. J., et al.
1987a The Spanish DIS: Reliability and concordance with clinical diagnoses in Puerto Rico. *Archives of General Psychiatry.* 44(8):420–426.

———, et al.
1987b The prevalence of alcohol abuse and dependence in Puerto Rico. In M. Gaviria and J. A. Arana, eds., *Health and Behavior: Research Agenda of Hispanics.* Chicago: University of Illinois at Chicago, Simon Bolívar Hispanic American Research and Training Program; pp. 127–144.

Carpenter, W., T. McGlashan, and J. Strauss
1977 The treatment of acute schizophrenia without drugs. *American Journal of Psychiatry* 134:14–20.

Carr, J.
1978 Ethnobehaviorism and the culture-bound syndromes: The case of amok. *Culture, Medicine and Psychiatry* 2:269–293.

———, and P. Vitaliano
1985 Theoretical implications of converging research on depression and culture-bound syndromes. In A. Kleinman and B. Good, eds., *Culture and Depression.* Berkeley: University of California Press; pp. 244–266.

Carstairs, M., and R. Kapur
1976 *The Great Universe of Kota: Change and Mental Disorder in an Indian Village.* Berkeley: University of California Press.

Castel, R., F. Castel, and A. Lovell
1982 *The Psychiatric Society.* New York: Columbia University Press.

Cawte, J.
1974 *Medicine Is the Law: Studies in Psychiatric Anthropology of Australian Tribal Societies.* Honolulu: University of Hawaii Press.

Centers for Disease Control (CDC)
    1984   *Morbidity and Mortality Weekly Report* 36(27), Table V, July 17.
Chatel, J., and R. Peele
    1971   The concept of neurasthenia. *International Journal of Psychiatry* 9:36–49.
Cheng, N.
    1987   *Life and Death in Shanghai.* New York: Grove Press.
Cheung, F., et al.
    1981   Somatization among Chinese depressives in general practice. *International Journal of Psychiatry in Medicine* 10:361–374.
Chrisman, N.
    n.d.   Popular culture explanatory models in primary care. (unpublished manuscript)
Clark, M., et al.
    1987   Hormones. *Newsweek,* Jan. 12, 53–59.
Clausen, J. A.
    1985   *The Life Course: A Sociological Perspective.* Englewood Cliffs, N.J.: Prentice-Hall.
Clayton, P. J.
    1974   Mortality and morbidity in the first year of widowhood. *Archives of General Psychiatry* 125:747–750.

——
    1979   The sequelae and nonsequelae of conjugal bereavement. *American Journal of Psychiatry* 136:1530–1543.

——
    1982   Bereavement. In E. S. Paykel, ed., *Handbook of Affective Disorders.* London: Churchill Livingstone.
Cleary, P.
    1987   Conceptualizing and measuring social support. In H. B. Weiss and F. Jacobs, eds. *Evaluating Family Processes.* Chicago: Aldine.
Clifford, J., and G. Marcus, eds.
    1986   *Writing Culture.* Berkeley: University of California Press.
Cohen, S., and S. L. Syme
    1985   *Social Support and Health.* New York: Academic Press.
Collis, R. J. M.
    1966   Physical health and psychiatric disorders in Nigeria. *Transactions of the American Philosophical Society,* New Series 56(4):1–45.
Comaroff, J.
    1985   *Body of Power, Spirit of Resistance.* Chicago: University of Chicago Press.
Connor, L.
    1982   Ship of fools and vessels of the divine. *Social Science and Medicine* 16:783–792.
Cooper, J., and N. Sartorius,
    1977   Cultural and temporal variations in schizophrenia. *British Journal of Psychiatry* 130:50–55.

Coyne, J.
　　1976　Toward an interactional description of depression. *Psychiatry* 39:28–
　　　　40.

――――, et al.
　　1981　Depression and coping in stressful episodes. *Journal of Abnormal Psy-*
　　　　chology 90:437–439.

Crapanzano, V.
　　1973　*The Hamadsha: A Study in Moroccan Ethnopsychiatry.* Berkeley:
　　　　University of California Press.

Csordas, T.
　　1984　The rhetoric of transformation in ritual healing. *Culture, Medicine*
　　　　and Psychiatry 7:333–376.

――――
　　1987　Health and the holy in African and Afro-American spirit possession.
　　　　Social Science and Medicine 24(1):1–11.

Day, R., et al.
　　1987　Stressful life events preceding the acute onset of schizophrenia. *Cul-*
　　　　ture, Medicine and Psychiatry 11:123–206.

Dean, S., and D. Thong
　　1972　Shamanism versus psychiatry in Bali. *American Journal of Psychiatry*
　　　　129:59–62.

DeVries, M., et al., eds.
　　1983　*The Use and Abuse of Medicine.* New York: Praeger.

Dimsdale, J., ed.
　　1980　*Survivors, Victims and Perpetrators: Essays on the Nazi Holocaust.*
　　　　Washington, D.C.: Hemisphere.

Dobkin de Rios, M.
　　1981　*Saladerra*—a culture-bound misfortune syndrome in the Peruvian
　　　　Amazon. *Culture, Medicine and Psychiatry* 5:193–213.

Dohrenwend, B.
　　1966　Social status and psychological disorder. *American Sociological Re-*
　　　　view 31:14–34.

――――, and B. Dohrenwend
　　1974　Social and cultural influences on psychopathology. *Annual Review of*
　　　　Psychology 25:417–452.

Doi, T.
　　1986　*The Anatomy of Self: The Individual Versus Society.* Tokyo: Kodan-
　　　　sha International.

Donzelot, J.
　　1980　The Policing of Families. New York: Pantheon.

Douglas, M.
　　1970　The healing rite. *Man* 5:302–308.

Dow, J.
　　1986　Universal aspects of symbolic healing: A theoretical synthesis. *Ameri-*
　　　　can Anthropologist 88(1):56–69.

Dressler, W.
    1985   Psychosomatic symptoms, stress and modernization. *Culture, Medi-
           cine and Psychiatry* 9(3):257–294.

Drinka, G. G.
    1984   *The Birth of Neurosis: Myth, Malady and the Victorians.* New York:
           Simon & Schuster.

DSM-III
    1980   Washington, D.C.: American Psychiatric Association Press.

Dull, J.
    1975   Implications of Chinese history for comparative studies of medicine
           in society. In A. Kleinman et al., eds., *Medicine in Chinese Cultures.*
           Washington, D.C.: USGPO for NIH; pp. 669–678.

Durkheim, E.
    1951   *Suicide.* Translated by J. A. Spaulding and G. Simpson. New York:
           The Free Press. (First edition 1897).

Durlak, J. A.
    1979   Comparative effectiveness of paraprofessional and professional
           helpers. *Psychological Bulletin* 86:80–92.

Ebigbo, P. O.
    1982   Development of a culture specific (Nigeria) screening scale of somatic
           complaints indicating psychiatric distress. *Culture, Medicine and Psy-
           chiatry* 6:29–44.

Edgerton, R.
    1967   *The Cloak of Competence.* Berkeley: University of California Press.

    ——

    1984   Anthropology and mental retardation. *Culture, Medicine and Psychi-
           atry* 8:25–48.

Egdell, H. G., and I. Kolven
    1972   Childhood hallucinations. *Journal of Child Psychology and Psychiatry*
           13:279–287.

Egeland, J. A.
    1986   Cultural factors and social stigma for manic-depression. *American
           Journal of Social Psychiatry* 6(4):279–286.

——, et al.
    1987   Bipolar affective disorders linked to DNA markers on chromosome 11.
           Nature 325:783–784, Feb. 26.

Eisenberg, D.
    1985   *Encounters with Qi.* New York: Norton.

Eisenberg, L.
    1980   What makes persons "patients" and patients "well"? *American Jour-
           nal of Medicine* 69:277–286.

    ——

    1984   Rudolph Virchow, where are you now that we need you? *American
           Journal of Medicine* 77:524–532.

————
1986   Mindlessness and brainlessness in psychiatry. *British Journal of Psychiatry* 148:497–508.

————
1987   Preventing mental, neurological and psychosocial disorders. *World Health Forum* 8(2):245–253.

————, and A. Kleinman, eds.
1981   *The Relevance of Social Science for Medicine*. Dordrecht, Holland: D. Reidel.

Eisenbruch, M.
1986   Cultural bereavement among Cambodian unaccompanied minors. *Community Health Studies* 9:313–314.

Eliade, M.
1964   *Shamanism: Archaic Techniques of Ecstasy*. New York: Pantheon.

Elliott, G. R., and C. Eisdorfer
1982   *Stress and Human Health: Analysis and Implications of Research. A Study of the Institute of Medicine, National Academy of Sciences*. New York: Springer.

Engel, G.
1980   The clinical application of the biopsychosocial model. *American Journal of Psychiatry* 137:535–544.

Escobar, J., et al.
1983   Depressive symptomatology in North and South American patients. *American Journal of Psychiatry* 140:47–51.

Estroff, S.
1981   *Making It Crazy*. Berkeley: University of California Press.

Fabrega, H.
1987   Psychiatric diagnosis: A cultural perspective. *Journal of Nervous and Mental Disease* 175(7):383–394.

————, and D. Silver
1973   *Illness and Shamanistic Curing in Zinacantan*. Stanford, Calif.: Stanford University Press.

Falloon, I., et al.
1982   Family management in the prevention of exacerbation of schizophrenia. *New England Journal of Medicine* 306:1437–1440.

Favazza, A., and M. Oman
1977   *Anthropological and Cross-Cultural Themes in Mental Health*. Columbia: University of Missouri Press.

————, and A. Faheem
1982   *Themes in Cultural Psychiatry: An Annotated Bibliography*. Columbia: University of Missouri Press.

Feinstein, A.
1987   The intellectual crisis in clinical science. *Perspectives in Biology and Medicine* 30(2):215–230.

Ferguson, D. M., and L. Horwood
  1984 Life events and depression in women. *Psychological Medicine* 14:881–890.

Field, M. D.
  1958 *Search for Security: An Ethno-Psychiatric Study in Rural Ghana.* London: Faber & Faber.

Finkler, K.
  1983 *Spiritist Healers in Mexico.* New York: Bergin & Garvey.

———
  1985 Symptomatic differences between the sexes in rural Mexico. *Culture, Medicine and Psychiatry* 9:27–58.

Fiske, D., and R. Shweder, eds.
  1986 *Metatheory in Social Science.* Chicago: University of Chicago Press.

Fortes, M., and D. Y. Mayer
  1969 Psychosis and social change among the Tallensi of Northern Ghana. In S. H. Foukes and G. S. Prince, eds., *Psychiatry in a Changing Society.* London: Tavistock.

Foucault, M.
  1966 *Madness and Civilization.* New York: Mentor.

Fox, R.
  1980 The evolution of medical uncertainty. *Milbank Memorial Fund Quarterly* 58(1):1–49.

Frank, J.
  1974 *Persuasion and Healing.* New York: Schocken (First edition 1961).

Freeman, H.
  1984 The scientific background. In H. Freeman, ed., *Mental Health and the Environment.* London: Churchill Livingstone.

Freidson, E.
  1986 *Professional Powers.* Chicago: University of Chicago Press.

Frese, M.
  1987 Alleviating depression in the unemployed. *Social Science and Medicine* 25(2):213–216.

———, and G. Mohr
  1987 Prolonged unemployment and depression in older workers. *Social Science and Medicine* 25(2):173–178.

Freud, S.
  1905 *On Psychotherapy.* In *Standard Edition of the Complete Psychological Works of Sigmund Freud, Vol. 7.* Translated by J. Strachey. London: Hogarth Press; pp. 257–268.

Gaines, A.
  1979 Definitions and diagnoses: Cultural implications for psychiatric help seeking and psychiatrists' definitions of the situation in psychiatric emergencies. *Culture, Medicine and Psychiatry* 3:381–418.

——
1982 Cultural definitions, behavior and the person in American psychiatry. In A. Marsella and G. White, eds., *Cultural Conceptions of Mental Health and Therapy*. Dordrecht, Holland: D. Reidel Publishing Co.

——, and P. Farmer
1986 Visible saints: Social cynosures and dysphoria in the Mediterranean tradition. *Culture, Medicine and Psychiatry* 10:295–330.

Garrison, V.
1977 The "Puerto Rican Syndrome" in psychiatry and espiritismo. In V. Crapanzano and V. Garrison, eds., *Case Studies in Spirit Possession*. New York: Wiley; pp. 383–448.

Gaviria, M., et al.
1984 Developing instruments for cross-cultural research. Paper presented at the American Psychiatric Association Annual Meeting.

Gaw, A., ed.
1982 *Cross-Cultural Psychiatry*. Boston: John Wright.

Geertz, C.
1973 *The Interpretation of Culture*. New York: Basic Books.

——
1984 Anti anti-relativism. *American Anthropologist* 86(2):263–348.

Giddens, A.
1986 *The Constitution of Society*. Berkeley: University of California Press.

Glick, L. B.
1967 Medicine as an ethnographic category: The Gimi of the New Guinea highlands. *Ethnology* 6:31–56.

Goffman, E.
1963 *Stigma*. Englewood Cliffs, N.J.: Prentice-Hall.

Goleman, D.
1985 Social workers vault into a leading role in psychotherapy: Psychiatrists and psychologists defend territory as competition increases. *Washington Post*, April 30.

——
1986 Psychiatry: First guide to therapy is fiercely opposed. *The New York Times*, September 23, p. C1.

Good, B.
1977 The heart of what's the matter: The semantics of illness in Iran. *Culture, Medicine and Psychiatry* 1:25–28.

——, et al.
1982 Toward a meaning centered analysis of popular illness categories. In A. Marsella and G. White, eds., *Cultural Conceptions of Mental Health and Therapy*. Dordrecht, Holland: D. Reidel; pp. 141–166.

——, M. J. D. Good, and R. Moradi
1985 The interpretation of Iranian depressive illness. In A. Kleinman and B. Good, eds., *Culture and Depression*. Berkeley: University of California Press; pp. 369–428.

———, and A. Kleinman
1985 Culture and anxiety. In A. H. Turns and J. P. Maser, eds., *Anxiety and the Anxiety Disorders*. Hillsdale, N.J.: Lawrence Earlbaum; pp. 297–324.

Goodman, N.
1978 *Ways of World Making*. New York: Hackett.

———
1984 Notes on the well-made world. *Partisan Review* 51(2):276–289.

Gould, S. J.
1987 Animals and us. *New York Review of Books* 34(11):20–25.

Gove, W. R., ed.
1975 *The Labeling of Deviance*. New York: Sage/Halstead.

Grob, G. N.
1986 Psychiatry and social activism: The politics of a speciality in post-war America. *Bulletin of the History of Medicine* 60:477–501.

Guarnaccia, P., et al.
In press *Nervios* in Puerto Ricans. *Medical Anthropology*.

Haberman, P. W.
1970 Ethnic differences in psychiatric symptoms reported in community surveys. *Public Health Reports* 85:495–502.

———
1976 Psychiatric symptoms among Puerto Ricans in Puerto Rico and New York City. *Ethnicity* 3:133–144.

Hadley, S., and H. D. Strupp
1976 Contemporary views of negative effects in psychiatry. *Archives of General Psychiatry* 33:1291–1302.

Hahn, R., and A. Gaines, eds.
1984 *Physicians of Western Medicine*. Dordrecht, Holland: D. Reidel.

———, and A. Kleinman
1983 Belief as pathogen, belief as medicine. *Medical Anthropology Quarterly* 14(4):3,16–19.

———
1984 Biomedical practice and anthropological theory. *Annual Review of Anthropology* 12:305–333.

Hall, R. C. W., ed.
1980 *Psychiatric Presentations of Medical Illness*. New York: Spectrum.

Hanauske-Abel, H. M.
1986 From Nazi Holocaust to nuclear holocaust. *Lancet*, Aug. 2, 271–273.

Handelman, D.
1967 The development of a Washo shaman. *Ethnology* 6:444–464.

Haracz, J.
1982 The dopamine hypothesis: An overview of studies with schizophrenic patients. *Schizophrenic Bulletin* 8(3):438–469.

Harding, C. M., et al.
    1987   The Vermont longitudinal study of patients with severe mental illness. Parts 1 and 2. *American Journal of Psychiatry* 144:718–726, 727–735.

Harkness, S.
    1987   The cultural mediation of postpartum depression. *Medical Anthropology Quarterly*, New Series 1:194–209.

Harner, M., ed.
    1973   *Hallucinogens and Shamanism*. New York: Oxford University Press.

Harwood, A.
    1977   Puerto Rican spiritism. Parts 1 and 2. *Culture, Medicine and Psychiatry* 1:69–97, 135–154.

———, ed.
    1981   *Ethnicity and Medical Care*. Cambridge, Mass.: Harvard University Press.

Havens, L.
    1985   *Making Contact*. Cambridge, Mass.: Harvard University Press.

Headley, L. A., ed.
    1983   *Suicide in Asia and the Near East*. Berkeley: University of California Press.

Heath, D.
    1986   Drinking and drunkenness in transcultural perspectives. Parts 1 and 2. *Transcultural Psychiatry Research Review* 23:7–42, 103–126.

Helman, C.
    1981   "Tonic," "Fuel" and "Food": Social and symbolic aspects of the long term use of psychotropic drugs. *Social Science and Medicine* 15B:521–33.

    1984   *Culture, Health and Disease*. Boston: John Wright.

    1985   Psyche, soma and society: The social construction of psychosomatic disease. *Culture, Medicine and Psychiatry* 9:1–26.

Henderson, A. S.
    1981   Social relationships, adversity and neurosis. *British Journal of Psychiatry* 138:391–398.

    1982   The significance of social relationships in the etiology of neuroses. In C. M. Pakes and J. Stevenson-Hurde, eds., *The Place of Attachment in Human Behavior*. New York: Basic Books.

———, and P. A. P. Moran
    1983   Social relationships during the onset and remission of neurotic symptoms. *British Journal of Psychiatry* 143:462–472.

———, et al.
    1986   Social support, dementia and depression among the elderly in Hobart. *Psychological Medicine* 16:1–10.

Herink, R.
  1980   *The Psychotherapy Handbook*. New York: New American Library.

Higginbotham, N.
  1984   *Third World Challenge to Psychiatry: Culture Accommodation and Mental Health Care*. Honolulu: East-West Center, University of Hawaii Press.

Hofer, M. A.
  1984   Relationships as regulators: A psychobiological perspective on bereavement. *Psychosomatic Medicine* 46(3):183–197.

Hofstadter, L.
  1987   Once bitten. *Stanford Medicine*, Winter, 23–25.

Hogarty, G. E., and S. Goldberg
  1973   Collaborative study group: Drug and sociotherapy in the aftercare of schizophrenic patients. *Archives of General Psychiatry* 28:54–64.

Holden, C.
  1986   Depression research advances, treatment lags. *Science* 233:723–726.

Hoosain, R.
  1986   Perception. In M. Bond, ed., *The Psychology of the Chinese People*. Hong Kong: Oxford University Press; pp. 38–72.

Horowitz, M.
  1976   *Stress Response Syndromes*. New York: Jason Aronson.

Horton, R.
  1967   African traditional thought and Western science, 1. *Africa* 37:50–71.

Hsieh, A., and J. Spence
  1982   Suicide and the family in pre-modern China. In A. Kleinman and T. Y. Lin, eds., *Normal and Abnormal Behavior in Chinese Culture*. Dordrecht, Holland: D. Reidel; pp. 29–48.

Hsu, F. L. K.
  1971   Psychosocial homeostasis and *Jen American Anthropologist* 73:23–44.

Jackson, S.
  1985   Acedia: The sin and its relationship to sorrow and melancholia. In A. Kleinman and B. Good, eds., *Culture and Depression*. Berkeley: University of California Press; pp. 43–62.

———
  1986   *Melancholia and Depression: From Hippocratic Times to Modern Times*. New Haven: Yale University Press.

Jacobson, D.
  1987a   Models of stress and meanings of unemployment. *Social Science and Medicine* 24(1):13–21.

———
  1987b   The cultural context of social support and support networks. *Medical Anthropology Quarterly*, New Series 1(1):42–67.

James, W.
　　1890　The hidden self. *Scribner's Magazine* 7:373.

Janes, C. R., et al., eds.
　　1986　*Anthropology and Epidemiology.* Dordrecht, Holland: D. Reidel.

Janzen, J.
　　1978　*The Quest for Therapy in Lower Zaire.* Berkeley: University of California Press.

Jaurès, J.
　　1986　1897 statement cited in J. D. Bredin, *The Affair: The Case of Alfred Dreyfus.* New York: Braziller.

Jegede, R. O.
　　1978　Outpatient psychiatry in an urban clinic in a developing country. *Social Psychiatry* 13:93–98.

Jencks, C.
　　1987　Genes and crime. *New York Review of Books* 34(2):33–40, Feb. 12.

Jenkins, J. H.
　　In press　Conceptions of schizophrenia as a problem of nerves: A cross-cultural comparison of Mexican-Americans and Anglo-Americans. *Social Science and Medicine.*

Jilek, W. G.
　　1974　*Salish Indian Mental Health and Culture Change.* Toronto: Holt, Rinehart and Winston of Canada.

――――
　　1982　*India Healing.* Blaine, Washington: Hancock House Publishers.

―――― and L. Jilek-Aall
　　1970　Transient psychosis in Africans. *Psychiatric Clinics* 3:337–364.

Jilek-Aall, L., et al.
　　1978　Sex role, culture and psychopathology: A comparative study of three ethnic groups in western Canada. *Journal of Psychological Anthropology* 6(4):473–488.

Joelson, L., and L. Wahlquist
　　1987　The psychological meaning of job insecurity and job loss. *Social Science and Medicine* 25(2):179–182.

Johnson, D., and C. Johnson
　　1965　Totally discouraged: A depressive syndrome of the Dakota Sioux. *Transcultural Psychiatry Research Review* 2:141–143.

Johnson, T., and A. Kleinman
　　1984　Cultural concerns in psychiatric consultation. In F. Guggenheim and M. Weiner, eds., *Manual of Psychiatric Consultation and Emergency Care.* New York: Jason Aronson; pp. 275–284.

――――
　　In press　Cultural factors in the medical interview. In M. Lipkin et al., eds., *The Medical Interview.* New York: The Task Force on the Medical Interview, Society of General Internal Medicine.

Jones, E. E.
    1986   Interpreting interpersonal behavior: The effect of expectancies. *Science* 234:41–46.

Jones, I., and D. Horne
    1973   Diagnosis of psychiatric illness among tribal aborigines. *Medical Journal of Australia* 1:345–349.

Kakar, S.
    1982   *Shamans, Mystics and Doctors.* New York: Knopf.

Kapferer, B.
    1983   *A Celebration of Demons: Exorcism and the Aesthetics of Healing in Sri Lanka.* Bloomington: Indiana University Press.

Kaplan, H.
    1983   *Psychosocial Stress: Trends in Theory and Research.* New York: Academic Press.

Kapur, M., et al.
    1979   *Psychotherapeutic Processes.* Bangalore, India: National Institute of Mental Health and Neurosciences.

Karno, M., et al.
    1987   Mental disorder among Mexican Americans and non-Hispanic whites in Los Angeles. In M. Gaviria and J. D. Arana, eds., *Health and Behavior: Research Agenda for Hispanics.* Chicago: University of Illinois at Chicago, Simon Bolívar Hispanic Research Program; pp. 110–126.

———, J. Jenkins, et al.
    1987   Expressed emotion and schizophrenic outcome among Mexican-American families. *Journal of Nervous and Mental Disease* 175:143–151.

Karasu, T. B.
    1986   The specificity versus non-specificity dilemmas: Toward identifying therapeutic change agents. *American Journal of Psychiatry* 143:687–694.

Katon, W., and A. Kleinman
    1981   Doctor-patient negotiation. In L. Eisenberg and A. Kleinman, eds., *The Relevance of Social Science for Medicine.* Dordrecht, Holland: D. Reidel.

———, et al.
    1982   Depression and somatization. Parts 1 and 2. *American Journal of Medicine* 72:127–135, 241–247.

———, et al.
    1984   The prevalence of somatization in primary care. Parts 1 and 2. *Comprehensive Psychiatry* 25(2):208–215, (3):305–314.

Katz, R.
    1982   *Boiling Energy: Community Healing Among the Kalahari Kung.* Cambridge, Mass.: Harvard University Press.

Kaufert, J., and W. W. Koolage
    1984   Role conflict among "culture brokers": The experience of native Canadian medical interpreters. *Social Science and Medicine* 18(3):283–286.

————, et al.
1985   Culture brokerage and advocacy in urban hospitals: The impact of Native language interpreters. *Santé, Culture, Health* 3(2):3–9.

Kearney, R., and B. Miller
1985   The spiral of suicide and social change in Sri Lanka. *Journal of Asian Studies* 45:81–101.

Kelso, D., and C. Attneave
1981   *Bibliography of North American Indian Mental Health.* Westport, Conn.: Greenwood Press.

Kendler, K. S., et al.
1984   A family history study of schizophrenia-related personality disorders. *American Journal of Psychiatry* 141:424–427.

Kennedy, J.
1987   *The Flower of Paradise: The Institutionalized Use of the Drug Qat in North Yemen.* Dordrecht, Holland: D. Reidel.

Kiev, A.
1972   *Transcultural Psychiatry.* Harmondsworth, England: Penguin.

Kinzie, D., et al.
1982   Development and validation of a Vietnamese language depression rating scale. *American Journal of Psychiatry* 139:1276–1281.

Kirmayer, L.
1984   Culture, affect and somatization. Parts 1 and 2. *Transcultural Psychiatry Research Review* 21(3):159–188, (4):237–262.

Kitaro, N.
1970   *Fundamental Problems of Philosophy: The World of Action and the Dialectical World.* Translated by D. A. Dilworth. Tokyo: Sophia University.

Klein, D., et al.
1983   Treatment of phobias II. Behavior therapy and supportive psychotherapy: Are there any specific ingredients? *Archives of General Psychiatry* 40:139–148.

Kleinman, A.
1977   Depression, somatization and the new cross-cultural psychiatry. *Social Science and Medicine* 11:3–10.

————
1980   *Patients and Healers in the Context of Culture.* Berkeley: University of California Press.

————
1982   Neurasthenia and depression. *Culture, Medicine and Psychiatry* 6 (2):117–190.

————
1985   Some uses and misuses of social science in medicine. In D. Fiske and R. Shweder, eds., *Metatheory in Social Science.* Chicago: University of Chicago Press; pp. 222–245.

————
1986   *Social Origins of Distress and Disease: Depression, Neurasthenia and Pain in Modern China.* New Haven: Yale University Press.

——
1987   Anthropology and psychiatry. *British Journal of Psychiatry* 151:447–454.

——
1988a   A window on psychiatry and mental health in China. *American Scientist* 76(1):22–27.

——
1988b   *The Illness Narratives: Suffering, Healing and the Human Condition.* New York: Basic Books.

——, L. Eisenberg, and B. Good
1978   Culture, illness and care. *Annals of Internal Medicine* 12:83–93.

——, and L. H. Song
1979   Why do indigenous practitioners successfully heal: A follow-up study of indigenous practice in Taiwan. *Social Science and Medicine* 130:7–26.

——, and J. Gale
1982   Patients treated by physicians and folk healers: A comparative outcome study in Taiwan. *Culture, Medicine and Psychiatry* 6(4):405–423.

——, and B. Good, eds.
1985   *Culture and Depression.* Berkeley: University of California Press.

——, and J. Kleinman
1985   Somatization. In A. Kleinman and B. Good, eds., *Culture and Depression.* Berkeley: University of California Press; pp. 429–490.

Klerman, G. L.
1987   Quoted in *Psychiatric News*, May 15, 8.

——, et al.
1984   *Interpersonal Psychotherapy of Depression.* New York: Basic Books.

Knox, R. A.
1987   The baffling "chronic mono" syndrome. *Boston Globe*, Jan. 12, C47.

Kraus, R., and P. Bufler
1979   Sociocultural stress and the American Native in Alaska. *Culture, Medicine and Psychiatry* 3:111–153.

Krause, N., and L. G. Carr
1978   The effects of response bias in the survey assessment of the mental health of Puerto Rican migrants. *Social Psychiatry* 13:167–173.

Kunitz, S.
1983   *Disease Change and the Role of Medicine.* Berkeley: University of California Press.

Kuper, A.
1987   The invention of primitive society. Lecture presented to the Department of Anthropology, Harvard University, Apr. 6.

Laderman, C.
1986   The ambiguity of symbols in the structure of healing. *Social Science and Medicine* 24(4):293–301.

La Fontaine, J.
    1975   Anthropology. In S. Perlin, ed., *A Handbook for the Study of Suicide.* New York: Oxford University Press; pp. 77–92.

Lakoff, G., and M. Johnson
    1980   *Metaphors We Live By.* Chicago: University of Chicago Press.

Lambo, T.
    1955   The role of cultural factors in paranoid psychosis among the Yoruba. *Journal of Mental Science* 101:239–266.

    ——

    1962   Malignant anxiety. *Journal of Mental Science* 108:256–264.

    ——

    1974   Psychiatry in Africa. *Psychotherpy and Psychodynamics* 24:26–34.

    ——

    1982   Psychotherapy in Africa. In E. Angeloni, *Annual Editions: Anthropology 82/83.* New York: Guilford; pp. 164–168.

Langness, L. L.
    1965   Hysterical psychosis in the New Guinea highlands: A Bena Bena example. *Psychiatry* 28:259–277.

——, and G. Frank
    1985   *Lives: An Anthropological Approach to Biography.* Novato, Calif.: Chandler and Sharp.

——, and H. Levine, eds.
    1986   *Culture and Retardation.* Dordrecht, Holland: D. Reidel.

Lasch, C.
    1977   *Haven in a Heartless World: The Family Beseiged.* New York: Basic Books.

    ——

    1979   *The Culture of Narcissism.* New York: Norton.

Latour, B., and S. Woolgar
    1979   *Laboratory Life: The Social Construction of Scientific Facts.* Beverly Hills: Sage.

Lazare, A.
    1973   Hidden conceptual models in clinical psychiatry. *New England Journal of Medicine* 288:345–350.

Leff, J.
    1981   *Psychiatry Around the Globe.* New York: Marcel Dekker.

——, et al.
    1982   A controlled trial of social intervention in the families of schizophrenic patients. *British Journal of Psychiatry* 141:121–134.

——, et al.
    1983   Life events, relatives' expressed emotion and maintenance of neuroleptics in schizophrenic relapse. *Psychological Medicine* 13:799–780.

——, and C. Vaughn
    1985   *Expressed Emotion in Families.* New York: Guilford.

Leighton, A., et al.
    1963a   *The Character of Danger: Psychiatric Symptoms in Selected Communities.* Vol. III, *The Stirling County Study of Psychiatric Disorder and Sociocultural Environment.* New York: Basic Books.

————, et al.
1963b. *Psychiatric Disorder Among the Yoruba.* Ithaca, N.Y.: Cornell University Press.

————, et al.
1968 The therapeutic process in cross-cultural perspective. *American Journal of Psychiatry* 124:1171–1183.

Leighton, A.
1986 Psychiatric epidemiology and social psychiatry. *American Journal of Social Psychiatry* 6(4):221–226.

Leslie, C., ed.
1976 *Asian Medical Systems.* Berkeley: University of California Press.

Levi, L.
1984 *Stress in Industry.* Geneva: International Labor Office.

Lévi-Strauss, C.
1967 *Structural Anthropology.* New York: Doubleday.

LeVine, R. A.
1973 *Culture, Behavior and Personality.* Chicago: Aldine.

Levy, R.
1973 *Tahitians: Mind and Experience in the Society Islands.* Chicago: University of Chicago Press.

Lewis, G.
1975 *Knowledge of Illness in a Sepik Society.* London: Athlone Press.

Lewis, I. M.
1971 *Ecstatic Religion: An Anthropological Study of Spirit Possession and Shamanism.* Harmondsworth, England: Penguin.

Lewis, T.
1975 A syndrome of depression in Oglala Sioux. *American Journal of Psychiatry* 133(2):753–755.

Lewontin, R. C., S. Rose, and L. J. Kamin
1984 *Not in Our Genes.* New York: Pantheon.

Liang, H., and J. Shapiro
1983 *Son of the Revolution.* New York: Knopf.

Lifton, R. J.
1983 *The Broken Connection: On Death and the Continuity of Life.* New York: Basic Books.

————
1986 *The Nazi Doctors: Medical Killing and the Psychology of Genocide.* New York: Basic Books.

Like, R.
Ms. Medical Anthropology Bibliography for Family Physicians.

Lin, E. H. B.
1984 Intraethnic characteristics and patient-physician interaction: Cultural blind spot syndrome. *Journal of Family Practice* 16(1):91–98.

Lin, K. M.
  1979   Transcultural training experience of a psychiatrist from East Asia. In
         J. Carlton, ed., *Dimension of Social Psychiatry*. Princeton, N.J.: Sci-
         ence Press; pp. 337–349.
——, and A. Kleinman
  1981   Recent development of psychiatric epidemiology in China. *Culture,
         Medicine and Psychiatry* 5:135–143.
——, A. Kleinman, and T. Y. Lin
  1982   Overview of mental disorders in Chinese culture. In A. Kleinman and
         T. Y. Lin, eds., *Normal and Abnormal Behavior in Chinese Culture*.
         Dordrecht, Holland: D. Reidel.
——, et al.
  1986   Ethnicity and psychopharmacology. *Culture, Medicine and Psychi-
         atry* 10:151–166.
——, and A. Kleinman
  In press Psychopathology and clinical course of schizophrenia: A cross-
         cultural perspective. *Schizophrenia Bulletin*.
Lin, N., et al.
  1979   Social support, stressful life events and illness: A model and an empiri-
         cal test. *Journal of Health and Social Behavior* 20(1):108–119.
——, et al.
  1986   Modeling the effects of social support. In N. Lin et al., eds., *Social
         Support, Life Events and Depression*. New York: Academic Press.
Lin, T. Y., ed.
  In press Neurasthenia in East Asian societies. *Culture, Medicine and Psy-
         chiatry*.
——, et al.
  1969   Mental disorders in Taiwan 15 years later. In W. Caudell and T. Y.
         Lin, eds., *Mental Health in Asia and the Pacific*. Honolulu: East West
         Center Press; pp. 66–91.
——, et al.
  1978   Ethnicity and patterns of help seeking. *Culture, Medicine and Psychi-
         atry* 2:3–14.
——, and D. Lin
  1982   Alcoholism among the Chinese. *Culture, Medicine and Psychiatry*
         6:109–116.
——, and M. C. Lin
  1982   Love, denial and rejection: Responses of Chinese families to mental
         illness. In A. Kleinman and T. Y. Lin, eds., *Normal and Abnormal
         Behavior in Chinese Culture*. Dordrecht, Holland: D. Reidel; pp.
         387–401.
Lipton, J., and J. Marbach
  1986   Ethnicity and the pain experience. *Social Science and Medicine*
         19:1279–1298.
Littlewood, R.
  1986   Cultural psychiatry in Britain today. *Curare* 9(1):9–16.
——, and M. Lipsedge
  1987   The butterfly and the serpent: Culture, psychopathology and biomed-
         icine. *Culture, Medicine and Psychiatry* 11:289–336.

Lock, M.
    1980   *East Asian Medicine in Urban Japan.* Berkeley: University of California Press.

    1986   Ambiguities of aging: Japanese experience and perception of menopause. *Culture, Medicine and Psychiatry* 10:23–46.

    1987   Protests of a good wife and wise mother: Somatization and medicalization in modern Japan. In M. Lock and E. Norbeck, eds., *Health and Medical Care in Japan.* Honolulu: University of Hawaii Press; pp. 130–157.

Low, S.
    1985   *Nervios in Costa Rica.* Philadelphia: University of Pennsylvania Press.

Luborsky, L., B. Singer, and L. Luborsky
    1975   Comparative studies of psychotherapies: Is it true that "everyone has won and all must have prizes"? *Archives of General Psychiatry* 32:995–1008.

——, et al.
    1985   Therapist success and its determinants. *Archives of General Psychiatry* 42:602–611.

Lumsden, D. P., ed.
    1984   *Community Mental Health Action.* Ottawa: Canadian Public Health Association.

Lutz, C.
    1985   Depression and the translation of emotional worlds. In A. Kleinman and B. Good, eds., *Culture and Depression.* Berkeley: University of California Press; pp. 63–100.

——, and G. White
    1986   The anthropology of emotions. *Annual Review of Anthropology* 15:405–436.

Macpherson, C., and L. Macpherson
    1987   Towards an explanation of recent trends in suicide in Western Samoa. *Man* 22(2):305–330.

Manschreck, T.
    1978   The atypical psychoses. *Culture, Medicine and Psychiatry* 2:233–268.

——, and A. Kleinman, eds.
    1977   *Renewal in Psychiatry: A Critical Rational Perspective.* Washington, D.C.: Hemisphere-Halsted.

    1979   Psychiatry's identity crisis: A critical rational remedy. *General Hospital Psychiatry* 1(2):166–173.

Manson, S., ed.
    1982   *New Directions in Prevention Among American Indian and Alaska Native Communities.* Portland: National Center for American Indian and Alaska Native Mental Health Research at the Oregon Health Sciences University.

——, et al.
   1985   The depressive experience in American Indian communities. In
          A. Kleinman and B. Good, eds., *Culture and Depression*. Berkeley:
          University of California Press; pp. 331–368.
Marsella, A.
   1979   Depressive experience and disorder across cultures. In H. Triandis and
          J. Draguns, eds., *Handbook of Cross-Cultural Psychology*. Vol. 6.
          Boston: Allyn & Bacon; pp. 237–290.
——, and G. White, eds.
   1982   *Cultural Conceptions of Mental Health and Illness*. Dordrecht, Hol-
          land: D. Reidel.
——, et al.
   1985   Cross-cultural studies of depressive disorders. In A. Kleinman and
          B. Good, eds., *Culture and Depression*. Berkeley: University of Cali-
          fornia Press; pp. 299–324.
Matchett, N. F.
   1972   Repeated hallucinatory experiences as part of the mourning process
          among Hopi Indian women. *Psychiatry* 35:185–194.
Mayr, E.
   1981   *The Growth of Biological Thought*. Cambridge, Mass.: Harvard Uni-
          versity Press.
McCormick, J. S.
   1986   Diagnosis: The need for demystification. *Lancet*, Dec. 20/27, 1434–
          1435.
McCreery, J. L.
   1979   Potential and effective meaning in therapeutic ritual. *Culture, Medi-
          cine and Psychiatry* 3:53–72.
McDermott, W., et al.
   1972   Health care experiment at Many Farms. *Science* 175:23–28.
McGoldrick, M., et al., eds.
   1982   *Ethnicity and Family Therapy*. New York: Guilford.
McGrath, G., and K. Lowson
   1986   Assessing the benefits of psychotherapy: An economic approach. *Brit-
          ish Journal of Psychiatry* 150:65–71.
McGuire, M. B.
   1983   Words of power: Personal empowerment and healing. *Culture, Medi-
          cine and Psychiatry* 7:221–240.
McHugh, P., and A. Slavney
   1986   *The Perspectives of Psychiatry*. Baltimore: Johns Hopkins University
          Press.
McHugh, S., and T. M. Vallis, eds.
   1986   *Illness Behavior*. New York: Plenum.
McKeown, T.
   1976a *The Modern Rise of Population*. New York: Academic Press.

   1976b *The Role of Medicine*. London: Nuffield Provincial Hospitals Trust.

   1980   *The Role of Medicine*. Princeton, N.J.: Princeton University Press.
Mechanic, D., ed.
   1982   *Symptoms, Illness Behavior and Help Seeking*. New Brunswick, N.J.:
          Rutgers University Press.

———, ed.
   1983   *Handbook of Health, Health Care and the Health Professions.* New York: Free Press.

———
   1986   Role of social factors in health and well being: Biopsychosocial model from a social perspective. *Integrative psychiatry* 4:2–11.

Messing, S.
   1986   Interdigitation of mystical and physical healing in Ethiopia. *Behavioral Science Notes* 3:87–104.

Métraux, A.
   1959   *Voodoo in Haiti.* New York: Oxford University Press.

Mezzich, J., and E. Raab
   1980   Depressive symptomatology across the Americas. *Archives of General Psychiatry* 37:818–823.

Minuchin, S., et al.
   1978   *Psychosomatic Families.* Cambridge, Mass.: Harvard University Press.

Mishler, E.
   1984   *The Discourse of Medicine: Dialectics of Medical Interviews.* Norwood, N.J.: Ablex.

———, et al.
   1981   *Social Contexts of Health, Illness and Patient Care.* London and New York: Cambridge University Press.

Mitchell, T., et al.
   1985   The DIS in Latin America. Paper presented at Annual Meeting of the American Psychiatric Association.

Moerman, D. E.
   1979   Anthropology of symbolic healing. *Current Anthropology* 20(1):59–80.

Moore, B.
   1970   *Reflections on the Causes of Human Misery.* Boston: Beacon Press.

———
   1978   *Injustice: The Social Basis of Obedience and Revolt.* New York: Sharpe.

———
   1987   *Authority and Inequality.* New York: Oxford University Press.

Moscicki, E. K., et al.
   1987   The Hispanic health and nutrition examination survey: Depression among Mexican Americans, Cuban Americans, and Puerto Ricans. In M. Gaviria and J. D. Arana, eds., *Health and Behavior: Research Agenda for Hispanics.* Chicago: University of Illinois at Chicago, Simon Bolívar Hispanic American Research Program; pp. 149–154.

Moser, K. A., et al.
   1986   Unemployment and mortality. *Lancet* 1:365–367.

Mulkay, M.
   1981   Action and belief or scientific discourse? *Philosophy of the Social Sciences* 11:163–171.

Mullings, L.
1984 *Therapy, Ideology and Social Change: Mental Healing in Urban Ghana.* Berkeley: University of California Press.

Mumford, E., et al.
1984 A new look at evidence about reduced cost of medical utilization following mental health treatment. *American Journal of Psychiatry* 141:1145–1158.

Munikata, T.
1986 Sociocultural background of the mental health system in Japan. *Culture, Medicine and Psychiatry* 10:351–366.

——— 1987 Japanese attitudes toward mental illness and mental health care. In T. S. Lebra and W. P. Lebra, eds., *Japanese Culture and Behavior.* Revised edition. Honolulu: University of Hawaii Press.

Murphy, H. B. M.
1968 Cultural factors in the genesis of schizophrenia. In D. Rosenthal and S. Kety, eds., *The Transmission of Schizophrenia.* Elmsford, N.Y.: Pergamon.

——— 1982 Comparative Psychiatry: The International and Intercultural Distribution of Mental Illness. New York: Springer-Verlag.

———, and A. C. Raman
1971 Chronicity of schizophrenia in indigenous tropical peoples. *British Journal of Psychiatry* 118:489–497.

Murphy, J.
1964 Psychotherapeutic aspects of shamanism on St. Lawrence Island, Alaska. In A. Kiev, ed., *Magic, Faith and Healing.* New York: Macmillan.

——— 1976 Psychiatric labeling in cross-cultural perspective. *Science* 191:1019–1028.

——— 1982 Cultural shaping and mental disorders. In W. R. Gove, ed., *Deviance and Mental Illness.* Beverly Hills: Sage; pp. 49–82.

Myers, J. K., et al.
1984 Six-month prevalence of psychiatric disorders in three communities. *Archives of General Psychiatry* 41:959–967.

Nash, J.
1967 The logic of behavior: Curing in a Maya Indian town. *Human Organization* 26:132–140.

Nations, M., et al.
1985 "Hidden" popular illnesses in primary care: Residents' recognition and clinical implications. *Culture, Medicine and Psychiatry* 9:223–240.

Navarro, V.
1986 *Crisis, Health and Medicine.* London: Tavistock.

Needham, R., ed.
1979 *Right and Left: Essays on Dual Symbolic Classification.* Chicago: University of Chicago Press.

Neki, J.
    1973   Guru-chela relationship: The possibility of a therapeutic paradigm.
            American Journal of Orthopsychiatry 43:755–766.

Ness, R.
    1980   The impact of indigenous healing activity: An empirical study of two
            fundamentalist churches. *Social Science and Medicine* 14B:167–180.

Newton, F., et al.
    1982   *Hispanic Mental Health Research: A Reference Guide.* Berkeley: Uni-
            versity of California Press.

Nichter, M.
    1981   Negotiations of the illness experience. *Culture, Medicine and Psychi-
            atry* 5:5–24.

    ——

    1982   Idoims of distress. *Culture, Medicine and Psychiatry* 5:379–408.

Oakeshott, M.
    1978   *Experience and Its Modes.* London: Cambridge University Press; pp.
            162–163. (First edition 1933).

Obeyesekere, G.
    1985   Depression, Buddhism and the work of culture in Sri Lanka. In
            A. Kleinman and B. Good, eds., *Culture and Depression.* Berkeley:
            University of California Press; pp. 134–152.

Ohnuki-Tierney, E.
    1984   *Illness and Culture in Contemporary Japan.* London: Cambridge
            University Press.

O'Nell, T.
    In press   Psychiatric investigations among American Indians and Alaska Na-
            tives: A critical review. *Culture, Medicine and Psychiatry.*

Opler, M. K., ed.
    1959   *Culture and Mental Health.* New York: Macmillan.

Orley, J., and J. Wing
    1979   Psychiatric disorders in two African villages. *Archives of General Psy-
            chiatry* 36:513–520.

Osterweis, M., et al.
    1984   *Bereavement.* Washington, D.C.: National Academy Press.

    ——, et al., eds.
    1987   *Pain and Disability.* Washington, D.C.: National Academy Press.

Parkes, C. M.
    1985   Bereavement. *British Journal of Psychiatry* 146:11–17.

Parloff, M. B., et al.
    1978   Research on therapist variables in relation to process and outcome. In
            S. Garfield and A. E. Bergin, eds., *Handbook of Psychotherapy and
            Behavior Change.* New York: Wiley.

Parsons, C.
    1985   Idioms of distress: Kinship and sickness in Tonga. *Culture, Medicine
            and Psychiatry* 8:71–94.

Paykel, E.
1978 Contribution of life events to causation of psychiatric illness. *Psychological Medicine* 8:245–253.

——, et al.
1969 Life events and depression. *Archives of General Psychiatry* 21:753–760.

Pentony, P.
1981 *Models of Influence in Psychotherapy.* New York: Free Press.

Pina-Cabral, J.
1986 *Sons of Adam, Daughters of Eve: The Peasant Worldview of the Alto Minho.* London: Oxford University Press.

Plessner, H.
1970 *Laughing and Crying: A Study of the Limits of Human Behavior.* Evanston, Ill.: Northwestern University Press.

Pope, H. G.
1986 Frequency and presentation of neuroleptic malignant syndrome. *American Journal of Psychiatry* 143(10):1222–1233.

Prince, R.
1968 Changing picture of depressive syndromes in Africa. *Canadian Journal of African Studies* 1:177–192.

——, ed.
1982 Shamans and endorphins. *Ethos* 10(4):299–423.

——, and F. Tcheng-Laroche
1987 Culture-bound syndromes and international classification of disease. *Culture, Medicine and Psychiatry* 11(1):3–20.

Racy, J.
1980 Somatization in Saudi women. *British Journal of Psychiatry* 137:212–216.

Raffel, S.
1979 *Matters of Fact: A Sociological Inquiry.* London: Routledge & Kegan Paul.

Rao, A. V.
1973 Depressive illness and guilt in Indian culture. *Indian Journal of Psychiatry* 15:231–236.

———
1984 Depressive illness in India. *Indian Journal of Psychiatry* 26:301–311.

Regier, D., et al.
1978 The defacto U.S. mental health service system. *Archives of General Psychiatry* 35:685–693.

Reid, J.
1983 *Sorcerers and Healing Spirits: Continuity and Change in an Aboriginal Medical System.* Canberra: Australian National University Press.

——, and T. Strong.
1987 *Torture and Trauma: The Health Care Needs of Refugee Victims in New South Wales.* Sydney: Cumberland College of Health Sciences.

Reiman, E. M., et al.
  1984   A focal brain abnormality in panic disorder. *Nature* 310:683–685.

Reiss, D.
  1981   *The Family Construction of Reality.* Cambridge, Mass.: Harvard University Press.

Reynolds, D.
  1976   *Morita Psychotherapy.* Berkeley: University of California Press.

———
  1983   *Naikan Psychotherapy: Meditation for Self-Development.* Chicago: University of Chicago Press.

Rhodes, L.
  1984   "This will clear your mind": The use of metaphors for medication in psychiatric settings. *Culture, Medicine and Psychiatry* 8:49–70.

Rin, H., and T. Y. Lin
  1962   Mental illness among Formosan aborigines as compared with Chinese in Taiwan. *Journal of Mental Science* 108:134–146.

Rioch, M. J.
  1966   Changing concepts in the training of therapists. *Journal of Consulting Psychology* 30(4):290–292.

Robert Wood Johnson Foundation
  1987   *Access to Health Care in the U.S.: Results of a 1986 Survey. Special Report #2.* Princeton, N.J.: R. W. Johnson Foundation.

Roberts, R. E.
  1980   Reliability of CES-D Scale in different ethnic groups. *Psychiatric Research* 2:125–134.

Robertson, M.
  1987   Molecular genetics of the mind. *Nature* 325:755, Feb. 26.

Robins, L. N., et al.
  1984   Lifetime prevalence of specific psychiatric disorders in three communities. *Archives of General Psychiatry* 41:949–958.

Rosaldo, M.
  1980   *Knowledge and Passion: Ilongot Notions of Self and Social Life.* London: Cambridge University Press.

Rose, N.
  1986   Psychiatry: The discipline of mental health. In P. Miller and N. Rose, eds., *The Powers of Psychiatry.* Cambridge, England: Polity Press; pp. 43–84.

Rose, R., Hurst, M., and A. Herd
  1979   Cardiovascular and endocrine responses to work and the risk of psychiatric symptoms in air traffic controllers. In J. Barrett, ed., *Stress and Mental Disorder.* New York: Raven Press.

Rosen, G., and A. Kleinman
  1984   Social science in the clinic: Applied contributions from anthropology to medical teaching and patient care. In J. Carr and H. Dengerink, eds., *Behavioral Science in the Practice of Medicine.* New York: Elsevier Biomedical.

Rosenberg, C.
  1962 The place of G. M. Beard in nineteenth century psychiatry. *Bulletin of the History of Medicine* 36:245-259.

Rosenfield, I.
  1986 Neural Darwinism: A new approach to memory and perception. *New York Review of Books* 33(15):21-279.

Rubel, A., et al.
  1984 *Susto.* Berkeley: University of California Press.

Rubinstein, D. H.
  1985 Suicide in Micronesia. In F. Hezel, D. Rubinstein, and G. White, eds., *Culture, Youth and Suicide in the Pacific: Papers from an East-West-Center Conference.* Honolulu: University of Hawaii Working Papers Series.

Rush, A. J., et al.
  1977 Comparative efficacy of cognitive therapy and pharmacotherapy in the treatment of depressed outpatients. *Cognitive Therapy and Research* 1:17-37.

Rutter, M.
  1986 Meyerian psychobiology, personality development and the role of life experiences. *American Journal of Psychiatry* 143:1077-1087.

———, and N. Madge
  1976 *Cycles of Disadvantage: A Review of Research.* London: Heinemann Educational.

Rycroft, C.
  1986 *Psychoanalysis and Beyond.* Chicago: University of Chicago Press.

Sahlens, M.
  1976 *Culture and Practical Reason.* Chicago: University of Chicago Press.

Salan, R., and T. Maretzki
  1984 Mental health services and traditional healing in Indonesia. *Culture, Medicine and Psychiatry* 7:377-412.

Sartorius, N. and A. Jablensky
  1976 Transcultural studies of schizophrenia. *WHO Chronicle* 30:481-485.

———, et al.
  1983 *Depressive Disorders in Different Cultures.* Geneva: WHO.

———et al.
  1986 Early manifestation and first contact incidence of schizophrenia. *Psychological medicine* 16:909-928.

Sasaki, Y.
  1969 Psychiatric study of the shamans in Japan. In W. Caudill and T. Y. Lin, eds., *Mental Health Research in Asia and the Pacific.* Honolulu: East-West Center Press.

Satter, D.
  1987 A test case: Anatoly Koryagin. *New York Review of Books* 34(2):3, Feb. 12.

Scheff, T.
  1979 *Catharsis in Healing, Ritual and Drama.* Berkeley: University of California Press.

Scheper-Hughes, N.
1979   *Saints, Scholars and Schizophrenics: Mental Illness in Rural Ireland.*
         Berkeley: University of California Press.

_____
1987   "Mental" in "Southie": Individual, family and community responses
         to psychosis in South Boston. *Culture, Medicine and Psychiatry* 11:53–
         78.

Schieffelin, E.
1976   *The Sorrow of the Lonely and the Burning of the Dancers.* New York:
         St. Martin's.

_____
1985   The cultural analysis of depressive affect: An example from New
         Guinea. In A. Kleinman and B. Good, eds., *Culture and Depression.*
         Berkeley: University of California Press; pp. 101–133.

Schwab, J. J.
1986   Psychiatric epidemiology. *American Journal of Social Psychiatry*
         6(4):215–220.

Schwartz, B.
1986   *The Battle for Human Nature.* New York: Norton.

Scull, A., ed.
1981   *Madhouses, Mad-Doctors, and Madmen: The Social History of Psy-
         chiatry in the Victorian Era.* Philadelphia: University of Pennsylvania
         Press.

Sebok, T. A.
1986   The doctrine of signs. *Journal of Social and Biological Structures*
         9(4):345–352.

Seligman, M.
1975   *Helplessness.* San Francisco: Freeman.

Sethi, B. B., et al.
1973   Depression in India. *Journal of Social Psychology* 91:3–13.

Shacter, S., and J. Singer
1962   Cognitive, social and physiological determinants and emotional
         states. *Psychological Review* 69:379–399.

Shapiro, A. K.
1959   The placebo effect in the history of medical treatment. *American
         Journal of Psychiatry* 16:298–304.

Shore, J., and S. Manson
1983   American Indian psychiatric and social problems. *Transcultural Psy-
         chiatry Research Review* 20(3):152–168.

Shorter Oxford English Dictionary
1967   Oxford: Clarendon Press. Third Edition.

Shweder, R. A.
1985   Menstrual pollution, soul loss and the comparative study of emotions.
         In A. Kleinman and B. Good, eds., *Culture and Depression.* Berkeley:
         University of California Press; pp. 182–215.

————, G. Miller
1986 The social construction of the person. In K. J. Gerger and K. E. Davis, eds., *The Social Construction of the Person.* New York: Springer-Verlag; pp. 40–69.

Sicherman, B.
1977 The uses of diagnosis: Doctors, patients and neurasthenics. *Journal of the History of Medicine and Allied Sciences* 32(1):33–54.

Sikanerty, R., and W. W. Eaton
1984 Prevalence of schizophrenia in the Labadi district of Ghana. *Acta Psychiatrica Scandinavica* 6:156–161.

Simons, R., and C. Hughes, eds.
1985 *The Culture-Bound Syndromes.* Dordrecht, Holland: D. Reidel.

Smilkstein, G., et al.
1981 Clinical social science conference. *Journal of Family Practice* 12 (2):347–353.

Smith, M., G. Glass, and T. Miller.
1980 *The Benefit of Psychotherapy.* Baltimore: Johns Hopkins University Press.

Snow, L.
1974 Folk medical beliefs and their implications for care of patients. *Annals of Internal Medicine* 81:82–96.

————
1978 Sorcerers, saints and charlatans: Black folk healers in urban America. *Culture, Medicine and Psychiatry* 2:69–106.

Spiegel, J.
1976 Cultural aspects of transference and counter-transference revisited. *Journal of the American Academy of Psychoanalysis* 4(4):447–467.

Srole, L., et al.
1962 *Mental Health in the Metropolis: The Midtown Manhattan Study.* New York: McGraw-Hill.

Staiano, K. V.
1986 *Interpreting Signs of Illness: A Case Study in Medical Semiotics.* New York: Mouton de Gruyter.

Starr, Paul
1983 *The Social Transformation of American Medicine.* New York: Basic Books.

Stevens, J.
1984 Brief psychosis: Do they contribute to the good prognosis and equal prevalence of schizophrenia in developing societies? *British Journal of Psychiatry* 151:393–396.

Stevens, W.
1972 The man with the blue guitar. In W. Stevens: *The Palm at the End of the Mind.* Edited by H. Stevens. New York: Vintage Books; pp. 133–149. (Originally published in 1937).

Stone, A. A.
    1987   The Japanese psychiatric scandal. *Boston Globe*, May 31, A26.

Stone, D.
    1984   *The Disabled State*. Philadelphia: Temple University Press.

Strupp, H. H., S., Hadley, and B. Gomes-Schwartz
    1977   *Psychotherapy for Better or Worse*. New York: Jason Aronson.

———, and S. Hadley
    1979   Specific versus non-specific factors in psychotherapy. *Archives of General Psychiatry* 36:1125–1136.

Sullivan, M.
    1986   In what sense is contemporary medicine dualistic? *Culture, Medicine and Psychiatry* 10:331–350.

Summerlin, F., ed.
    1980   *Religion and Mental Health: A Bibliography*. Washington, D.C.: USGPO for National Institute of Mental Health.

Tambiah, S. J.
    1968   The magical power of words. *Man* 3:175–208.

    1977   The cosmological and performative significance of a Thai cult of healing. *Culture, Medicine and Psychiatry* 1:97–132.

    1985   *Culture, Thought, and Social Action*. Cambridge, Mass.: Harvard University Press.

Taussig, M.
    1980   *The Devil and Commodity Fetishism in South America*. Chapel Hill: University of North Carolina Press.

    1987   *Shamanism, Colonialism and the Wild Man: A Study in Terror and Healing*. Chicago: University of Chicago Press.

Taylor, E.
    1984   *William James on Exceptional Mental States. The 1896 Lowell Lectures*. Amherst: University of Massachusetts Press; p. 140.

Teja J. S., et al.
    1971   Depression across cultures. *British Journal of Psychiatry* 119:253–260.

Tennant, C.
    1983   Life events and psychological morbidity. *Psychological Medicine* 13:483–486.

Thompson, D., and D. Goldberg
    1987   Hysterical personality disorder. *British Journal of Psychiatry* 150:241–245.

Thurston, A.
    1987   *Enemies of the People*. New York: Knopf.

Tiger, L.
    1979   *Optimism: The Biology of Hope*. New York: Touchstone.

Torgerson, S.
    1984   Genetic and nosological aspects of schizotypal and borderline personality disorders. *Archives of General Psychiatry* 41:546–554.

Torrey, E. F.
  1980   *Schizophrenia and Civilization.* New York: Jason Aronson.

———
  1986   *Witchdoctors and Psychiatrists: The Common Roots of Psychotherapy and Its Future.* New York: Harper & Row.

Torrey, E. F., et al.
  1984   Endemic psychosis in western Ireland. *American Journal of Psychiatry* 141:966–969

Townsend, J. M.
  1978   *Cultural Conceptions of Mental Illness.* Chicago: University of Chicago Press.

Tripp-Reimer, T., and P. Brink
  1985   Culture brokerage. In G. Bulechek and J. McCloskey, eds., *Nursing Interventions.* Philadelphia: Saunders; pp.352–364.

Truax, C. B., and R. R. Carkhoff
  1962   *Toward Effective Counseling and Psychotheray.* Chicago: Aldine.

Tseng, W. S., J. McDermott, and T. W. Maretzki, eds.
  1974   *People and Cultures in Hawaii.* Honolulu: University of Hawaii Press.

Turner, B.
  1985   *The Body and Society.* Oxford: Basil Blackwell.

Turner, V.
  1967   *The Forest of Symbols.* Ithaca, N.Y.: Cornell University Press.

———, and E. M. Bruner, eds.
  1986   *The Anthropology of Experience.* Urbana: University of Illinois Press.

Tyrer, P.
  1986   New rows of neuroses: Are they an illusion? *Integrative Psychiatry* 4:25–31.

Uhlenhuth, G., and D. Duncan
  1968   Subjective change with medical student therapists: Some determinants of change in psychoneurotic outpatients. *Archives of General Psychiatry* 18:532–540.

Vaughn, C., and J. Leff
  1976   The measurement of expressed emotion in the families of psychiatric patients. *British Journal of Social and Clinical Psychology* 15:157–165.

Vernon, S., et al.
  1982   Response tendencies, ethnicity and depression scores. *American Journal of Epidemiology* 116:482–495.

Wallace, A. F. C.
  1959   The institutionalization of cathartic and control strategies in Iroquois religious psychotherapy. In M. K. Opler, ed., *Culture and Mental Health.* New York: Macmillan.

Warner, R.
  1985   *Recovery from Schizophrenia: Psychiatry and Political Economy.* New York: Routledge & Kegan Paul.

Waxler, N.
    1977 Is outcome for schizophrenia better in non-industrialized societies. *Journal of Nervous and Mental Disease* 167:144–158.

———
    1981 Learning to be a leper. In E. Mischler et al., *Social Contexts of Health, Illness and Patient Care.* London: Cambridge University Press; pp. 169–194.

Weidman, H. H.
    1977 Falling out. *Social Science and Medicine* 13B:95–112.

———
    1978 *Miami Health Ecology Project Report, Volume 1: Ethnicity and Health.* Miami: University of Miami School of Medicine, Dept. of Psychiatry.

Weir, S.
    1980 *Qat in Yemen: Consumption and Social Change.* London: British Museum Publications.

Weisberg, D. H.
    1984 Physicians' private clinics in a northern Thai town. *Culture, Medicine and Psychiatry* 8:165–186.

———, and S. O. Long, eds.
    1984 Biomedicine in Asia. *Culture, Medicine and Psychiatry* 8(2):117–205.

Weiss, M.
    1985 The interrelationship of tropical disease and mental disorder. *Culture, Medicine and Psychiatry* 9:121–200.

———, et al.
    1986 Traditional concepts of mental disorder among Indian psychiatric patients. *Social Science and Medicine* 23:387–392.

———, and A. Kleinman
  In press Depression in cross-cultural perspective. In P. Dasein et al., eds., *Contributions of Cross-Cultural Psychology to International Mental Health.* New York: Plenum.

Weissman, M., and G. Klerman
    1977 Sex differences and the epidemiology of depression. *Archives of General Psychiatry* 34:98–111.

Werner, H., and B. Kaplan
    1967 *Symbol Formation.* New York: Wiley.

Westermeyer, J., and R. Wintrob
    1979 Folk criteria for the diagnosis of mental illness in rural Laos. *American Journal of Psychiatry* 136:755–761.

White, G.
    1982 The ethnographic study of cultural knowledge of mental disorder. In A. Marsella and G. White, eds., *Cultural Conceptions of Mental Health and Illness.* Dordrecht, Holland: D. Reidel; pp. 69–96.

———, and J. Kirkpatrick, eds.
    1985 *Person, Self and Experience: Exploring Pacific Ethnopsychologies.* Berkeley: University of California Press.

WHO
  1973   *The International Pilot Study of Schizophrenia.* Geneva: WHO.

———

  1979   *Schizophrenia: An International Follow-up Study.* Chichester: John Wiley & Sons.

Wig, N. N., et al.
  1987   Expressed emotional schizophrenia in North India, I. The cross-cultural transfer of ratings of relatives' expressed emotion. *British Journal of Psychiatry* 151:156–159.

Wikan, U.
  1980   *Life Among the Poor in Cairo.* London: Tavistock.

Williams, G. H., and P. H. N. Wood
  1986   Common sense beliefs about illness. *Lancet*, Dec. 20/27, 1435–1437.

Williams, J., and R. Spitzer
  1984   *Psychotherapy Research.* New York: Guilford.

Wing, J.
  1978   Social influences on the course of schizophrenia. In L. Wynne et al., eds., *The Nature of Schizophrenia.* New York: Wiley.

Wolpe, J.
  1958   *Psychotherapy by Reciprocal Inhibition.* Stanford, Calif.: Stanford University Press.

Wyatt, R. J. and E. G. De Renzo
  1986   Scienceless to homeless. (Editorial) *Science* 234:1309, 12 December.

Xu, J. M.
  1987   Some issues in the diagnosis of depression in China. *Canadian Journal of Psychiatry* 32(5):368–370.

Yang, K. S.
  1986   Personality. In M. Bond, ed., *The Psychology of the Chinese People.* New York: Oxford University Press; pp. 106–170.

Yeh, E. K., et al.
  1987   Social changes and prevalence of specific mental disorders in Taiwan. *Chinese Journal of Mental Health* 3(1):31–42.

Yelin, E., et al.
  1980   Toward an epidemiology of work disability. *Milbank Memorial Fund Quarterly* 58(3):386–414.

Young, A.
  1977   Order, analogy and efficacy in Ethiopian medical divination. *Culture, Medicine and Psychiatry* 1:183–200.

———

  1980   The discourse on stress and the reproduction of conventional knowledge. *Social Science and Medicine* 14B:133–146.

Yue, D. Y., and C. Wakeman
  1985   *To the Storm: The Odyssey of a Revolutionary Chinese Woman.* Berkeley: University of California Press.

Zborowski, M.
  1952   Cultural components in responses to pain. *Journal of Social Issues* 8:16–30.

———

  1969   *People in Pain.* San Francisco: Jossey-Bass.

Index

Printed in the United States
60276LVS00001B/256-339